The Truth Behind Hormone Replacement Therapy

What You Need to Know to Remain Youthful and Healthy

SELMA RASHID, M.D.

Publishing support provided by
Ignite Press
5070 N. Sixth St. #189
Fresno, CA 93710
www.IgnitePress.us

ISBN: 979-8-9868200-0-2
ISBN: 979-8-9868200-1-9 (Ebook)

For bulk purchase and for booking, contact:

Selma Rashid, M.D.
AntiAgingMedicalGroup.com

Library of Congress Control Number: 2022914740

Cover design by Divya Balu
Edited by Emma Hatcher
Interior design by Jetlaunch

FIRST EDITION

ACKNOWLEDGMENTS

For every woman who has been my patient, I am deeply and forever grateful. These bright, truth-seeking women have been my inspiration. Due to everything that they have shared with me, and by allowing me to help them, I gained experience that is not achievable by medical knowledge and scientific data alone.

Many of my patients were told by their doctors that they are simply getting old and should learn to accept the reality of aging. These women defied the comfort level of their primary care physicians and gynecologists and began to understand the logic of science and nature. They took a huge leap from what was "normal" and did what was intellectually sound. I admire their intellect and sense of discernment.

These women are true heroes for the next generation, because their sharing provides us with information that is otherwise unattainable. There will be no well-designed studies on the hormones our bodies make. Even if governments or private entities donated the funds for a well-designed (double-blind, placebo-controlled) study, it would be unethical and unrealistic to do a study comparing one group of women who take proper hormones versus another group who do not over the course of twenty to thirty years. Future generations of women will draw from the experiences of women such as my patients.

These women who placed their trust in me not only helped themselves and allowed me to increase my knowledge—their personal experiences and health benefits will help both current and future generations of women. To all these beautiful, amazing women, I am forever grateful.

I would like to thank Patricia Iyer, my editor, who went above and beyond to ensure my book is understandable by the lay person, without losing the essence of the message.

TABLE OF CONTENTS

Foreword. vii

Introduction. ix

Chapter 1: Controversies About Hormone
Replacement Therapy 1

Chapter 2: What Are Hormones,
and Why Do We Need Them?. 33

Chapter 3: Bioidentical and Synthetic Hormones—
Biochemistry Made Easy 43

Chapter 4: Estrogen. 53

Chapter 5: Progesterone. 59

Chapter 6: Estradiol and Progesterone Effects
On The Brain. 63

Chapter 7: Osteoporosis and Osteoarthritis. 79

Chapter 8: Skeletal Muscle, Tendons, and Ligaments 93

Chapter 9: Estradiol and Cardiovascular Health. 103

Chapter 10: Estradiol and Progesterone Effects
on the Immune System. 113

Chapter 11: Testosterone in Men. 125

Chapter 12: Prostate Cancer, BPH, and Testosterone 137

Chapter 13: Testosterone in Women 141

Chapter 14: Breast Cancer 145

Chapter 15: Thyroid Gland 157

Chapter 16: Adrenal Glands 165

Chapter 17: Growth Hormone 171

Conclusion 177

Endnotes 181

About the Author 209

FOREWORD

Would you like to live as fully and with as much health as possible as you age? It is hard to say no to that question. In fact, we spend billions of dollars per year on the desire to stay healthy for as long as we can.

Hormone replacement therapy is one of the tools available in the fight to remain healthy. It seems like it should be so simple. Once our body stops producing hormones at menopause or andropause, we can take artificially produced hormones and get the same benefits, right? You will find out why that is *not* correct.

Dr. Selma Rashid's book reveals that our hormones are far more complicated than we imagine. An intricate, intertwined connection of various types of hormones keeps us functioning. Every part of our bodies needs hormones.

In this carefully researched book, Dr. Rashid exposes the history behind decades of the efforts of healthcare professionals and scientists to explore the benefits of artificially produced hormones. Their theory was that it should be possible to create artificial hormones that would duplicate the benefits of naturally produced hormones. A great deal of time and money went into trying—and failing—to prove that fake hormones were just as good as the ones that your body produces.

The pharmaceutical industry generates huge profits by manufacturing synthetic hormones. They must be able to establish a patent on a drug to sell it. A bioidentical hormone (chemically the same as a naturally produced hormone) cannot be patented. When scientists were unable to verify the safety of fake hormones, the pharmaceutical industry turned to education and misinformation: let's encourage physicians and medical schools to see artificial hormones as useful and safe.

Dr. Rashid strips away the confusing information about manufactured hormones. When you read this book, you will understand the profit motives behind the relentless campaign to promote synthetic hormones. You will see that there is an alternative—safe, bioidentical hormones that treat menopause and andropause; minimize the problems of aging; and keep us healthy longer. And you will understand that taking fake hormones for bodybuilding or growth stimulation is a dangerous practice with big risks.

After reading this book, you will walk away with a greater appreciation for the complexity of our bodies and the power of tools to help us gracefully age. Dr. Rashid lays it out in a carefully constructed way to explain the science and profit motives of hormone replacement therapy. The information in this book will help you make an informed decision about whether you should seek guidance for getting help with hormone replacement.

Knowing that bioidentical hormone therapy replacement is a choice will help in your own decision making.

As the editor of this book, it was my pleasure to work with Dr. Rashid to bring you this critical information so that you know the alternatives and can work with your healthcare provider to make the decisions best for you.

— Pat Iyer, MSN, RN

INTRODUCTION

BEYOND THE SYMPTOMS OF MENOPAUSE, EXTENSION OF YOUTH AND WELL-BEING WITH AGING

This book reveals the truths and facts that everyone should know about the aging process and the decisive role of correctly administered hormone replacement therapy in preventing age-related diseases, remaining healthy, and being fully functional through every decade of our lives.

The hormone story is not new. By the 1930s, medical professionals realized that the loss of estradiol was linked to osteoporosis (bone degeneration). Shortly afterward, research showed that cardiovascular disease increases with the decline in estradiol. Since then, thousands of studies have demonstrated the health benefits of estradiol and progesterone in women and testosterone in men. We now know that every function of the human system depends on these hormones' physiological (normal, healthy) levels.

Medical science and data support the replacement of estradiol and progesterone in women and testosterone in men. Still, it isn't easy to find healthcare providers who correctly practice bioidentical hormone replacement therapy (therapy with hormones identical to what the human body makes). Decades of high-profile studies on synthetic hormones produced by Big Pharma (pharmaceutical industry) resulted in bad outcomes. They created an environment of circulating misinformation, not clarifying the difference between synthetic and bioidentical hormones or the risks of taking hormones orally.

Some physicians believe that hormone replacement therapy is dangerous. This concern is rooted in faulty research. As you will read later in this book, researchers carried out extensive studies to determine the beneficial effects of synthetic hormones. The results of these studies showed that synthetic progesterone is associated with breast cancer. Oral synthetic estrogen is associated with an increased risk of blood clots.

The people involved in these studies were not just pharmaceutical companies, such as Wyeth (Big Pharma), but also staff of the most prestigious institutions in the country, including investigators from Harvard, Stanford, UCLA Medical Center, Fred Hutchinson Cancer Research Center, and over twenty other prestigious US medical institutions.[1] Not many physicians would remotely consider questioning the integrity of such studies.

Although performed with artificial hormones, the results of these studies were linked in people's minds with bioidentical hormones, which are not the same as synthetic hormones. These studies created confusion and misinformation about the safety of bioidentical hormones. To add to the damage, websites from some of these institutions continue to display misleading information about the safety of bioidentical hormones.

Menopause, Andropause, and the Symptoms of Low Hormones

Symptoms of menopause are only a warning sign of the onset of rapid aging and the degenerative process. Menopause and andropause (decline in testosterone with aging) are a transition phase from a healthy balanced state to a state of continuous degeneration that is due to loss of estradiol and progesterone in women and a decline of testosterone in men.

Typical symptoms of menopause include hot flashes, night sweats, foggy brain, mood changes, vaginal dryness, low libido, low energy, weight gain, poor sleep, and so on. Not all women have symptoms of menopause, and men don't have any noticeable signs of andropause (lowering testosterone production). However, everyone undergoes continuous degenerative processes after menopause and andropause.

Aging and the Degenerative Process

We have different expectations of individuals' physical and mental health and performance after we turn fifty years old. The quality of health dramatically changes every decade after age fifty. Although the degenerative process is continuous, the impact of the accumulated changes is more noticeable every decade.

We expect individuals approaching their eighties and above to have some dementia; a weaker neurological system; poorer balance; osteoporosis; osteoarthritis; significant changes in body composition (with more fat and less muscle); and degenerative joints, tendons, and ligaments. The respiratory, cardiovascular, digestive, and urological systems also deteriorate. We know that older individuals have weaker immune systems.

Individuals over sixty-five years old are at high risk for life-threatening complications from the flu and COVID-19 and are advised to get vaccines for influenza, COVID-19, pneumonia, and shingles. With every decade after fifty, the recovery from disease is slower and the accumulation of the chronic disease of aging increases.

Aging While Remaining Youthful

In this book, you will learn that aging with a completely different trajectory is possible. You can retain a healthy brain, nervous system, muscles, ligaments, joints, tendons, bones, sleep quality, mood, memory, cognition, sexual function, and libido and so much more once these hormones are in the correct physiological ranges. The degenerative process will be dramatically reduced by replacing estradiol and progesterone in women and testosterone in men to the levels produced by a healthy body in the late thirties.

The years beyond retirement should be the best years of our lives, where we are physically and mentally healthy and independent. We should be able to continue to enjoy life, enhanced by our accumulated knowledge and experiences. Instead, we suffer from age-related diseases and frailty, which are largely preventable. This book provides critically important information regarding the aging process that everyone should be aware of.

Why Hormone Replacement Therapy Is Not the Standard of Care

Most healthcare providers and lay people do not understand the impact on health and functionality due to the loss of estradiol and progesterone in women and testosterone in men. They are led to believe that aging and loss of estradiol, progesterone, and testosterone are normal and acceptable.

Yes, it is normal, but it should not be accepted and needs to be addressed. The medical and pharmaceutical industries make the most significant profit from treating the diseases of aging, not preventing them.

Big Pharma and Bioidentical Hormones

Our government protects us in many ways. Mainstream medicine does a beautiful job in treating disease. Big Pharma (the pharmaceutical industry) has also done incredible work over the decades and has produced numerous lifesaving drugs. But the picture isn't perfect. Bioidentical hormones (the hormones that a human body makes) are not patentable and, therefore, not profitable. Due to conflicts of interest, we have been denied the truth for many decades.

Big Pharma successfully convinced otherwise-accomplished physicians and other prescribers, such as nurse practitioners, that synthetic (fake) hormones are the same as—if not better than—what the human body makes (bioidentical). This campaign further jeopardized progress in recognizing the benefits of bioidentical hormones.

After synthetic hormones gained bad press, Big Pharma has been trying to reenter the hormone market with variations in the preparations of bioidentical hormones, where the patent is in the combinations, concentrations, and delivery method. They are making every effort to influence the Food and Drug Administration (FDA) and government to stop compounding pharmacies from making bioidentical hormones, so that they can once again control the market. Their efforts have potentially alarming consequences.

The Power and Influence of Big Pharma

Second only to mining and crude oil production, Big Pharma is the most profitable industry in the world and has powerful, far-reaching influences. Their impact on the FDA is awe-inspiring. Before 1992, the FDA was fully funded by taxpayer dollars. Since 1992, FDA's funding from Big Pharma has steadily increased and is reported to be about forty-five to fifty percent. As well as securing their influence on the FDA, Big Pharma substantially influences medical training programs and politicians. By allowing this to happen, the FDA is implicated in making deplorable decisions, which hurt patients the most.

It would be blissful if the government, the healthcare industry, and Big Pharma indeed always had our best interests at heart. In some cases, they do; but it is not always so. Big Pharma's influence over unethical policymakers has damaging consequences on our healthcare system that go far beyond the topic of hormone replacement therapy.

Here are a few consequences of Big Pharma's influence on the US government, politics, and the US healthcare system:

- Education about bioidentical hormone replacement therapy has been kept out of the medical curriculum for decades. Prescribers receive misinformation; they are not trained in or provided with the complete truth about hormone replacement therapy. As a result, the people they serve continue to suffer from preventable and age-related diseases, have a poorer quality of life, and are deprived of health and functionality in the last few decades of their lives.

- America ranks about thirty-fourth according to the Bloomberg Global Health Index. This ranking is tragically low, considering that the United States has the best-trained physicians and top medical technology in the world—a fact most recently displayed by the United State's response to the COVID-19 crisis.

- Prescription drugs are drastically more expensive in the US than anywhere else. As a result, many people continue to suffer and remain untreated or order medicines from other countries (in some cases, from third-world countries, which is at the risk of counterfeit medications).

- The US healthcare system is one of the worst in any developed nation. Access to medical care is insufficient and limited in outpatient medicine, especially for the poor, who typically come to the hospital only when their disease is out of control. Due to government policies, hospitals are required to treat these patients. Most of these patients either have no insurance or Medicaid, which means that the hospitals lose money. Consequently, the hospital billing departments recover costs from paying individuals by increasing the cost of healthcare, resulting in higher insurance premiums.

- The government subsidies to hospitals are insufficient. Additionally, due to the astronomically high cost of health insurance, many people are putting off their healthcare until they qualify for Medicare.

- After losing trust in the healthcare system, many people defer to alternative treatments, especially to treat cancer, which has led to tragic outcomes.

Hormone Therapy for the Prevention of Age-Related Degeneration

Due to public pressure, bioidentical hormone replacement therapy is gaining acceptance for menopausal symptom relief in newly menopausal women. There is still resistance toward (and no medical consensus for) treating women who wish to take hormone replacement to prevent chronic disease. This ignorance stems from senseless interpretations from flawed and harmful studies using synthetic hormones (which are NOT safely administered bioidentical hormones).

Andropause, a stage of aging for men that is due to low testosterone, results in a steady decline in testosterone, and there are no dramatic symptoms such as hot flashes or night sweats. Consequently (and unfortunately), men go through years of slow degeneration, deprived of critical therapy.

Although hormone replacement therapy is best started when hormone levels begin to decline to suboptimal ranges (typically, forty-five-plus years old), it is still not too late to prescribe bioidentical hormone replacement therapy. It can be beneficial even if patients are in their sixties and seventies. For the countless benefits of correctly administered hormone therapy, there is no reason to believe that we ever need to stop using bioidentical hormone replacement therapy.

What Can We Do?

We will inevitably age, but how we choose to age is our decision. We must evaluate all the pertinent information and facts to make this critically important decision. For decades, we have been misled and denied the truth, due to the conflicting interests of Big Pharma and the influence that they have on the healthcare industry and the government.

Without knowing how hormone replacement can help to dramatically reduce the chronic diseases and degenerative changes that are inevitable after menopause and andropause, we deprive ourselves of the most powerful therapy available to keep us as healthy and functional as possible throughout our life's last four to five decades. We have a solution to truly aging well and like never before, we should know all the pertinent medical information about it.

What You Will Learn

As a practicing physician, I wrote this book to unveil the knowledge that you need in order to enjoy a quality life. You will discover the role of hormones in your health as well as the differences between synthetic and bioidentical hormones. This book shares this knowledge so that you may make informed decisions about hormone use. Here is some important information you will take away:

1. Understanding the importance of hormones, what they are, and what they do.

2. Understanding the difference between bioidentical and synthetic hormones and the importance of bioidentical hormones.

3. Equipping yourself with the knowledge on why hormones became controversial so that when an unknowledgeable healthcare professional provides wrong information, you can have a meaningful discussion rather than be intimidated or confused.

4. If a healthcare professional states that estradiol, progesterone, or testosterone causes cancer (which is incorrect), you should ask for proof from the medical literature, not unsubstantiated opinion or hearsay.

5. Understanding why I recommend that you find a knowledgeable physician who is willing to balance your hormones safely and responsibly:

   a. Only bioidentical hormones should be used.

   b. Estradiol, progesterone, or testosterone should not be taken by mouth.

   c. Blood levels should be carefully monitored so that levels are in physiological (normal, healthy levels).

In over twenty years of practicing medicine, in addition to passionately devoting my time to bioidentical hormone replacement therapy for the prevention of age-related diseases, I also work as a hospital physician. One of the greatest regrets that I have when I see elderly patients is knowing how preventable their frailty, loss of function, and debility would have been if they had been provided the correct treatment a few decades earlier. Not many of my patients wish to live forever, but every one of them values health, well-being, and living in dignity above almost anything else. I see elderly couples battling age-related diseases with recurrent hospital and physician visits instead of enjoying their retirement after decades of hard work.

The three most significant reasons people are hesitant to start hormone replacement therapy are:

1. Being told that it is dangerous and linked to causing cancer (which is false),

2. Not understanding how hormones affect our health and well-being, and

3. Being unable to find a knowledgeable physician.

After you read this book, you will have a new perspective on the role of hormones in your health and an appreciation for the marvelous ways that our bodies function.

CONTROVERSIES ABOUT HORMONE REPLACEMENT THERAPY

Aging with Health, Vibrance, and Grace

Hormone balance is the essence of health and wellness. Women should live decades beyond menopause with health, energy, and vitality based on current medical knowledge. Women without underlying medical diseases and healthy lifestyles expect to live into their nineties.

Menopause—the Beginning of Accelerated Deterioration in Health

The average age of menopause is about fifty-one. In the period known as perimenopause, there is a noticeable decline in ovarian hormone production, starting about ten years before menopause. During perimenopause, many women begin having some of the symptoms of menopause but still have a regular menstrual cycle.

Menopause comes with numerous degenerative health changes, including (but not limited to):

- poor sleep quality,
- low energy,

- osteoporosis,
- decline in cognition and memory,
- depression,
- apathy,
- loss of muscle strength,
- cardiovascular issues such as hypertension and dyslipidemia,
- low sex drive,
- vaginal dryness,
- inability to lose weight, and
- skin and hair changes.

Not every woman has symptoms of menopause, such as hot flashes, night sweats, or mood changes, but every woman has continuous degeneration of health and wellness after menopause.

With the correct prescriptions, women can benefit from hormone replacement therapy throughout their lives. Many barriers stand in the way of achieving this goal, including misinformation, poorly designed studies, and the pressures of pharmaceutical companies.

Circulation of False Information

Controversies over hormone replacement therapy existed from at least the 1940s and peaked in 2002 with the release of the initial results of the **Women's Health Initiative study.**

One of the questions most frequently asked by patients that I'm aware of is, "How can a medical treatment so pivotal to our health be controversial and disregarded by most healthcare professionals?"

This chapter explains the last century's main events, which led to confusion and misinformation about hormone replacement therapy. It outlines the chain of events:

1. The discovery of hormones,
2. The immediate action of the pharmaceutical industry which made synthetic (fake) rather than real (bioidentical) hormones,
3. Multiple studies of synthetic hormones unsuccessfully trying to prove their benefits, and
4. The creation and circulation of misinformation about hormones.

200 BC—The Importance of Hormones Recognized

The recognition that hormones are vital to normal human functioning is centuries old. By around 200 BC, the Chinese isolated hormones from human urine and used them for medicinal purposes.

1025 AD—Menstrual Problems Treated with Hormones

By 1025 AD, the Chinese prepared extracts of male and female urine to treat menstrual cycle problems (dysmenorrhea) as well as other disorders including hypogonadism (failure of the testes to produce sufficient hormones) in men. Even hundreds of years before this, studies were being done on thyroid tissue.

1800s—Multiple Studies Were Taking Place

By 1855 in Europe, researchers conducted experiments on glands and the products they secreted. Numerous research centers were involved in understanding the effects and importance of hormones.

Around 1880, Robert Battey removed ovaries from women who had painful periods, abnormal bleeding, and other menstrual cycle problems. These same women developed symptoms of hot flashes and vaginal atrophy. Researchers realized that the ovaries made some substance that, when absent, created symptoms. In 1897, Herbert Fosbery used ovarian extracts to treat hot flashes. A few years later, Nicolas Gendrin proposed that menstruation was related to ovulation. In 1896, Emil Knauer from Vienna was experimenting with rabbit ovaries.

1900s—Estrogen Discovered

About 100 years ago, in the 1920s, staff of numerous laboratories in Europe simultaneously extracted estrogen from the urine of pregnant women, and, within a few years, several estrogen products were available. Clinicians recognized that estrogen blocked hot flashes. Over time, they noted that estrogen prevented bone loss and then discovered that giving estrogen prevents ovulation.

Isolation of Human Estrogen

In the United States, the FDA is responsible for protecting public health. They evaluate the safety of medications and medical devices and are the gatekeepers who control which medications reach the public. This is important when it comes to the topic of hormones, because many different types of estrogen exist in nature.

Women produce three types of estrogen: estrone, estradiol, and estriol. None of them is patentable, and they do not need FDA approval. On the other hand, the FDA has to approve use of any estrogen that a woman's body does not produce. Hormones made by a woman's body are called bioidentical. (See chapter 3 on bioidentical and synthetic hormones for more details.) Molecularly altered or different versions are called synthetic.

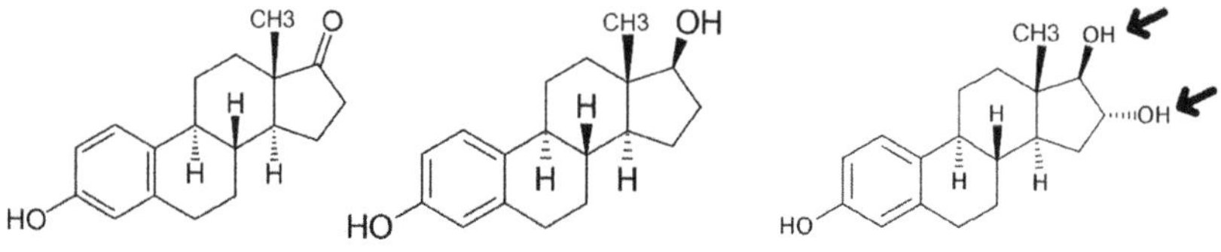

Diagram 1: The three types of bioidentical/human estrogens.

The First Bioidentical Estrogen—Emmenin

In the 1930s, a Canadian researcher, James Collip, extracted estrogen from the urine of pregnant women. The result was Emmenin, marketed by Ayerst. Emmenin mainly contained *estriol*, a metabolic byproduct of **estradiol** (the main estrogen made by the human ovary).

Introduction of Synthetic Estrogen

In 1941, the Canadian company, Ayerst, McKenna & Harrison, introduced Premarin®, a complex mixture of more than fifty different estrogens, derived from the urine of pregnant horses, also referred to as *conjugated equine estrogen* (CEE). The company merged with American Home products and became Wyeth. In 1942, the FDA approved Premarin® for the treatment of hot flashes and other menopausal symptoms.[2]

Premarin (also known as conjugated equine estrogen [CEE])

Premarin® is a synthetic product that contains estrogens that are quite different from the estrogen that a woman's body makes. Although this synthetic estrogen mix suited some women, it didn't help everyone, nor did it provide all the benefits of a woman's own (bioidentical) estrogen.

Oral Contraceptives

Shortly after Premarin® came into the market, clinicians realized that giving women estrogen prevented ovulation and found a new use for synthetic hormones. This discovery ultimately led to the sexual revolution: the ability to engage in sex without fearing pregnancy.

Enovid was the first birth control pill, composed of Mestranol and Norethynodrel (synthetic versions of estrogen and progesterone, respectively.) In June 1957, the FDA approved Enovid to treat menstrual disorders. In June 1960, FDA approved its use as a contraceptive.

By the 1960s, no one had done any significant studies on estrogen, progesterone, or synthetic versions, other than using Enovid on Puerto Rican women. The patients did not receive much information about the purpose of this study.

1960s—Blood Clots from Oral Estrogen Suspected

Within a few years of oral contraceptives being in the market, a physician who was head of the medical research council of the Great Britain Statistical Research Unit received alarming reports of otherwise healthy young women suffering from blood clots. The clots in the legs or lungs were presumed to be associated with oral contraceptives.

Frank Speizer and Martin Vessay, who were also working at the Great Britain Statistical Research Unit, were concerned that millions of healthy women were likely to be exposed to the risk of blood clots with no warning or plans for follow up. Speizer and Vessay suggested doing a long-term follow-up of a large group of women, to determine the safety of oral contraceptives.

In 1974, Speizer and Vessay received funding from the National Cancer Institute. They initially tried to recruit doctors' wives for the trial, but then realized that a group of women with stronger medical knowledge was needed. They shifted their attention on nurses, and launched their study, The Nurses' Health Study.

The Nurses' Health Study

The Nurses' Health Study had three parts. It was an uncontrolled study (a study where there is no comparison against another group) and required nurses to complete complex questionnaires every two years over a period of several years.

Part 1 conclusion

Data showed there was a higher risk of stroke, coronary heart disease, and breast cancer in patients on oral contraceptives. The risks reduced with time once a participant stopped taking the oral contraceptive.

Part 2 conclusion

Postmenopausal hormone therapy increased the risk of stroke and breast cancer.

Recently, menopausal women had a reduced risk of coronary heart disease.

The Nurses' Health Study initially gained tremendous attention; but later, researchers received a lot of criticism, mainly due to the way that the data was collected and interpreted.

Regardless of the criticism, the study did not significantly change the way that women were using birth control pills. Patients generally trusted their doctors, the pharmaceutical companies, the FDA, and the government. The package inserts included the associated risks, but not many people read or understood the risks, which is common even today.

Nurses' Health Study—Further Details

The study had three parts, led by three different primary investigators.

Part 1 began in 1976, led by Frank Speizer. About 121,700 married female nurses between the ages of thirty to fifty-five were recruited and provided biannual questionnaires. Seventy-one percent returned the questionnaires. The study investigated contraceptives, smoking, cancer, cardiovascular disease, and later added dietary questions.

Part 2, led by Walter Willett, began in 1989 and recruited about 116,430 nurses ages twenty-five to forty-two. The focus was women's health and oral contraceptives (including brand and length of use). Questions on exercise and food intake were later added.

Between 1996 and 1999, researchers collected blood and urine samples from about 30,000 nurses. About 18,500 gave two blood samples and one urine sample timed within the menstrual cycle.

Between 2010 and 2012, researchers gathered a second set of samples from about 16,500 of the same group of women who had reached menopause. The study included DNA from cheek cells in 2006.

Complex data collected every other year focused on employment status, shift work, family history of cancer, heart disease, and other diseases, reproductive history, menopause, medications, screening tests, leisure time, physical activity, sedentary time, sleep patterns, alcohol use, weight, height, body measurements, diet (including during adolescence), smoke exposure, living arrangements, neighborhood characteristics, environmental exposures, mental health, social networks, optimism skill, caregiving and caregiving stress, quality of life, and activities of daily living.

Part 3, led by Jorge Chavarro, began in 2010 with a target of 100,000 participants and is still ongoing. The focus is on dietary patterns, lifestyle, environment, new hormone preparations, and fertility/pregnancy, adolescent diet and breast cancer. Participants are between ages nineteen to forty-nine and include Canadians, different types of health workers, and males. Questionnaires are web-based.

A "Biological Revolution"

The 1960s were a thriving era for oral contraceptives and postmenopausal hormone replacement therapy. The pharmaceutical industry dominated the synthetic hormones market; there were no bioidentical hormones available.

In 1966, Dr. Robert A. Wilson, a British-born gynecologist who practiced in New York City, New York, published his book *Feminine Forever*, which became an international bestseller, further increasing the popularity of hormones. Wilson referred to hormone replacement therapy as the *biological revolution*.

Wilson believed that menopause was a hormone deficiency disease, curable and preventable by taking estrogen. Wilson presented hormone replacement therapy as the biological revolution, a treatment that could allow women to free themselves from the many negative effects of low estrogen and preserve femininity. He wrote, "Every woman alive today has the option of remaining feminine forever . . . It is simply no longer true that the sexuality of a woman past forty necessarily declines more rapidly than that of her husband." He paid special attention to the benefits of estradiol regarding osteoporosis, and overall femininity. He asserted, "Estrogen therapy doesn't change a woman. On the contrary—it keeps her from changing."

Wilson was also involved in a controlled study of 304 women ages forty to seventy taking hormone replacement therapy. The study, "The Roles of Estrogen and Progesterone in Breast and Genital Cancer," was published in the *Journal of American Medical Association* in 1962.[3]

Those who soaked up Wilson's advice had no idea that he had a motive for pushing synthetic hormones. Unfortunately, Wilson's popularity diminished after reports from the *New Republic* and *Washington Post* discovered documents showing that Wilson received payments for writing the book and for speaking *on behalf of companies making hormone replacement therapy*. After his son confirmed this, the drug companies had "no comments."

Introduction of Synthetic Progesterone

In the 1970s, research studies found that estrogen *without* progesterone ("unopposed estrogen") was associated with an *increased* risk of endometrial cancer. This news had a negative impact on hormone replacement therapy's reputation.[4, 5] Researchers later discovered that reducing the dose of estrogen and combining it with progesterone could *reduce* the risk of endometrial cancer,[6] leading to renewed interest in hormone replacement therapy (HRT). By this time, the FDA approved hormone replacement therapy to treat hot flashes and menopausal symptoms, but not for the prevention of chronic conditions.

Around 1986, Premarin® (synthetic estrogen) was prescribed for bone loss that was due to osteoporosis. There were talks in the medical industry that *every* postmenopausal woman should take Premarin® for the rest of her life.

In 1988, the FDA approved Premarin® use for prevention of osteoporosis.[7, 8] During the same time, many observational studies suggested that hormone replacement therapy had numerous benefits in the prevention of chronic diseases.[9, 10, 11, 12]

Synthetic Hormones for Chronic Diseases Prevention

Between the late 1980s and early 1990s, the American College of Physicians developed the first guidelines for using hormone replacement therapy as a preventive therapy for the chronic diseases of postmenopausal women.[13, 14] Again, only synthetic hormones were being used, however, this approval didn't last long.

1990s—A Thriving Era for Hormone Replacement Therapy

In the early 1990s, hormone replacement therapy (HRT) was at its all-time peak. Wyeth dominated the market with Premarin® (synthetic estrogen) and Provera® (synthetic progesterone).

Wyeth's influence on the FDA has historically been strong. A few other pharmaceutical companies tried to get into the hormone replacement therapy market by introducing generic versions of Premarin®. The problem of the emerging competition for Wyeth was resolved when the FDA concluded that generics were not interchangeable with Premarin. In 1991, the FDA withdrew approval of all other generic versions of Premarin®.

Concern About Cardiovascular Health and Hormones

Clinicians had some concerns about the possible impact of synthetic progesterone on the benefits seen with estrogen, particularly in respect to the cardiovascular system.[15] The results of the **Nurses' Health Study** claimed there were positive effects of estrogen and progesterone on cardiovascular health in newly menopausal women. Based on these claims, the FDA required that the presumed cardiovascular benefits of hormone replacement therapy be confirmed by randomized controlled clinical trials. This led to another study, the Heart and Estrogen/Progestin Replacement Study (HERS).

1992—The First Major Controlled Study on Hormone Replacement Therapy: The HERS Trial

The HERS trial study took place from July 1992 to July 2001. Its goal: to test the safety and efficacy of Premarin® (conjugated equine estrogen) and Provera® (medroxyprogesterone acetate)—a synthetic progesterone, for prevention of recurrent coronary heart disease (CHD) events in women with known coronary artery disease.

Results from the **HERS trial** *contradicted* the results of the **Nurses' Health Study.** To review, part one of the **Nurses' Health Study** concluded that there was a *higher* risk of stroke, coronary heart disease, and breast cancer when women took oral contraceptives, and the risk decreased after discontinuing the oral contraceptives. Part two concluded that postmenopausal women on hormone therapy had *an increased* risk of stroke and breast cancer and that recently menopausal women had a *reduced risk* of coronary heart disease.

Here's what the HERS trial concluded

- In women taking estrogen and progesterone, it showed a slight *increase* in heart disease in the first year, then a slight *decrease* in years three to five.
- The study did not measure breast cancer incidence.

HERS II: An extension of HERS trial

- The HERS II showed no cardiovascular benefits for women taking hormones.
- The cardiovascular benefits seen in years three to five of the HERS trial no longer existed in the HERS II trial.
- There were no reports of an increase in breast cancer.

When the results came out, people were neither clearly told that the hormones used in the HERS trial were synthetic hormones, nor that oral estrogen was a risk for blood clots.

HERS Trial—Further Details

The study took place between July 1992 and July 2001. It was a double-blind, placebo-controlled study involving 2,340 women with coronary artery disease and an intact uterus who were randomized to receive 0.625 mg/d conjugated estrogens and 2.5 mg daily of medroxyprogesterone acetate versus placebo.

Researchers studied myocardial infarction and coronary heart disease (CHD) death. In addition, they measured coronary artery bypass grafting heart revascularization, angina, serum lipids, quality of life, compliance, uterine bleeding or endometrial hyperplasia, vasomotor and genitourinary symptoms, adverse effects, thromboembolic events, symptomatic gallbladder disease, fractures, cancer, stroke, peripheral arterial disease, and total mortality.

This randomized, double-blind trial occurred with post-menopausal women with coronary artery disease. Its goal: to determine if estrogen and progestin alters the risk for CHD in postmenopausal women with established CHD. The participants included 2,340 women who had a uterus. The researchers wished to determine if those randomized to receive estrogen-progestin replacement therapy had the same frequency of CHD events (myocardial infarction and CHD death) as those randomized to placebo.

Participants were evaluated every four years. During an average follow-up of 4.1 years, results showed no overall reduction in coronary heart disease events among postmenopausal women with established CHD. However, the hormone group had an increased rate of thromboembolic events and gallbladder disease. There was a decreased risk of CHD in years three to five.

The HERS II trial enrolled 2,321 women from the HERS trial and was conducted at outpatient and community settings at twenty US clinical centers. Some of the participants had open label therapy at the discretion of their personal physicians. Women who took the hormones derived no significant benefit. Any benefit in years three to five from HERS trial was not demonstrated in the HERS II trial.

Although the HERS and HERS II trials did not report any negative findings regarding breast cancer, the news was worrisome regarding cardiovascular disease. The positive conclusion was that hormone therapy did not increase breast cancer.

All the studies so far had conflicting results regarding heart disease. Statistics of women in the population (epidemiologic data) showed that women had less heart disease than men before menopause. Still, after menopause, their rate of heart disease paralleled that of men.

Based on the knowledge of the effects of estrogen and progester-one produced by the human body, clinicians and researchers still believed that estrogen and progesterone were beneficial to the heart.

1995—Another Study to Prove Cardiac Benefits: PEPI Trial

Researchers were still trying to prove human cardiac benefits with non-human hormones. PEPI (postmenopausal estrogen/pro-gestin interventions) was a three-year, multicenter, randomized, double-blinded, placebo-controlled clinical trial. Researchers used different combinations of Premarin® (synthetic estrogen) and Provera® (synthetic progesterone).

Brief conclusions

- Some favorable effects on LDL cholesterol and fibrinogen were seen.

- Researchers did not evaluate the incidence of breast cancer.

PEPI Trial—Further Details

The PEPI study involved 847 healthy postmenopausal women ages forty-five to sixty-four. Its goal: to assess differences on heart disease risk factors (lipid metabolism, carbohydrate metabolism/serum insulin, coagulation/hemostasis) in women taking one of three regimens:

- Premarin®, also known as conjugated equine estro-gen (CEE), alone (0.625 mg), or

- placebo, or

- three different combinations of Premarin® with medroxyprogesterone acetate (MPA).

The three combinations were:

    a. CEE and MPA 10 mg on days one to twelve of the month

    b. CEE and MPA 2.5 mg daily

    c. CEE and MPA 200 mgs on days one to twelve.

Women taking CEE alone and with an intact uterus had the least success in following the medication schedule.

Results showed a favorable effect on LDL-cholesterol and fibrinogen. No significant effect on blood pressure or insulin was noted. The study did not evaluate the incidence of breast cancer. Women on CEE alone had greater endometrial hyperplasia (uterus lining thickening).

Around the same time, the British initiated the ambitious **Million Women Study**, focusing on the effects of hormone replacement therapy on women's health.

1996—Million Women Study

This was a British study that intended to analyze data from more than 1 million women aged fifty to sixty-four. The study was uncontrolled and relied on self-reported data. Dame Valerie Beral and the team of researchers at the Cancer Epidemiology Unit at Oxford University led the study, in collaboration with the Cancer Research UK and the National Health Service, and additional funding from the Medical Research Council (UK).

Million Women Study—Further Details

The key focus was to study the effects of hormone replacement therapy on women's health. Between 1996 and 2001, women ages fifty to sixty-four and over were invited to join the Million Women Study. They received an invitation to attend breast cancer screening at one of the sixty-six participating NHS breast cancer screening centers in the UK. At the centers, the women received the study questionnaire which they were requested to complete and return at the time of screening. About 70 percent of those attending the program returned the questionnaires.

The researchers studied these questions:

1. What effects do combined estrogen and progestin hormone therapy preparations have on breast cancer risk?

2. Are breast cancers detected at a screening in women who have used HRT or oral contraceptives different in size and invasiveness from cancer seen in women who have never used these hormones?

3. How does HRT use affect the efficacy of breast cancer screening?

4. How does HRT use affect mortality from breast cancer and other conditions?

Conclusions of the Million Women Study

The initial analysis received extensive press coverage. The results appeared to confirm preliminary findings from other studies:

- Women currently using progesterone-estrogen HRT were more likely to develop breast cancer than those not using HRT.

- The negative effect was substantially more significant for combined estrogen-progesterone than estrogen only.

- Current users of estrogen-progesterone HRT had a two-fold increased risk of developing breast cancer.

- Current use of estrogen-*only* had a 1.3 increased risk of developing breast cancer.

A reanalysis of the study, led by Samuel Shapiro and published in 2012, refuted the initial conclusion that HRT increased the risk of breast cancer. The authors claimed that the research had not in fact established a causal relationship between HRT and breast cancer and that the original analysis was flawed. Shapiro concluded that HRT may or may not increase the risk of breast cancer, but the Million Women Study did *not* establish that it does.

The article led by Samuel Shapiro asserted, "Despite the massive size of the Million Women Study, the findings for E+P (estrogen and progesterone) and ET (estrogen therapy) did not adequately satisfy the criteria of time order, information bias, detection bias, confounding, statistical stability and strength of association, duration-response, internal consistency, external consistency or biological plausibility. Had detection bias resulted in identifying women aged 50–55 years of 0.3 additional cases of breast cancer in ET users per 1000 per year, or 1.2 in E+P users, it would have nullified the apparent risks reported."[16]

1990s—No Consensus on a Public Health Policy

After decades of research, researchers could not achieve a consensus on hormone replacement therapy. Every controlled study used some combination of Premarin® (conjugated equine estrogen) and Provera® (medroxyprogesterone acetate). Other research (which was uncontrolled and relied on self-reported data) involved various preparations of *synthetic* hormones, mainly used for contraception.

The investigations could not provide a satisfactory answer to the repeatedly raised concern that, among postmenopausal women, cardiovascular disease, cancer, and osteoporosis were the leading cause of health problems and impaired quality of life; cardiovascular disease and cancer were the leading cause of death.

Researchers agreed that more testing through clinical trials should occur before establishing a public health policy with guidelines. With the domination of Big Pharma, specifically Wyeth, the focus remained on proving the benefits of synthetic hormones, *not* hormones naturally produced by the human body.

The Long Arm of the Pharmaceutical Industry

For decades, pharmaceutical companies dominated the field of medicine and have financially influenced the government and healthcare system—including medical schools and training programs. They sought to sway prescribers by subsidizing free cruises and lunches, paying authors of articles in journals (which touted the benefits of their medications), and giving free medication samples, pens, pads, and other benefits. They wielded their influence both in obvious and hidden ways.

The medically trained investigators involved in the studies ignored the obvious difference between real and fake hormones and pushed the interests of powerful pharmaceutical companies.

1998—The Women's Health Initiative Study (WHI)

This study is considered a landmark study—and it is the most extensive research of its kind. The investigation used synthetic hormones produced by Wyeth and changed how hormones were viewed for almost two decades. The announcement of the initial results in 2002 created mass confusion, panic, and fear. Hormone replacement became magnitudes more controversial.

The research was designed with the hypothesis that estrogen therapy would reduce coronary artery disease and osteoporosis-related fractures. Due to the concern over the relationship of hormone replacement with elevated breast cancer risk, breast cancer was selected as a *primary adverse outcome*. Additional outcomes monitored included stroke, pulmonary embolism, endometrial cancer, colorectal cancer, hip fracture, and death due to other causes.

Hormones used in the study:

Estrogen: Conjugated equine estrogen (CEE), also known as Premarin®—synthetic hormone.

Progesterone: Medroxyprogesterone acetate (MPA), also known as Provera®—synthetic hormone.

Prempro®: The combination of Premarin® and Provera®.

The study had two divisions:

1. Prempro® vs. placebo, given to women who had a uterus, and
2. Premarin® vs. placebo, given to women without a uterus.

Brief Overview of the WHI Study

In 1991, researchers announced plans to do the study and received a budget of $650 million from the government over fifteen years. Recruitment began in 1993, and the study finally started in 1998. Almost 28,000 postmenopausal women ages fifty to seventy-nine were recruited and managed in forty US clinical centers in twenty-three states.

The Fred Hutchinson Cancer Research Center gained the role of the WHI's Clinical Coordinating Center (CCC), which was responsible for maintaining consistency between the forty clinical centers and collecting, managing, and analyzing the data of the WHI study.

Here are the ages of the participants who took both estrogen and progesterone, what percentage of the participants were in this age group, and how many were in that group:

- Fifty to fifty-four = CEE (Estrogen) and MPA (Progesterone): 14 percent of participants (2,029 total people), CEE: 15 percent (1,396).

- Fifty to fifty-nine: CEE and MPA: 25 percent (3,492), CEE: 23 percent (1,916).

- Sixty to sixty-nine: CEE and MPA: 50 percent (7,512), CEE: 50 percent (4,852).

- Seventy to seventy-nine: CEE and MPA: 24 percent (3,574), CEE: 26 percent (2,575).

The combination division received CEE at a dose of 0.625 mg/day and MPA at a dose of 2.5 mg/day. They totaled 16,605. Some of the women took estrogen alone: they totaled 10,739. The estrogen-only division received CEE at a dose of 0.625 mg/day.

Again, note that:

Prempro® is a combination of Premarin® and Provera® = synthetic.

Premarin® is conjugated equine estrogen (CEE) = synthetic.

Provera® is Medroxyprogesterone acetate (MPA) = synthetic.

Results of the Women's Health Initiative study

2002—Initial Results of the Prempro® (CEE/MPA) Division

The trial was originally designed to last for nine years. However, when researchers looked at the data about 5.2 years after the study started, they found:

Prempro® group had an *increased* risk of breast cancer, coronary artery disease, stroke, and pulmonary embolism.

There were ethical issues involved in continuing a study when the results indicated possible harm associated with the medications. Therefore, researchers halted the study in July 2002. Restrictions on hormone replacement therapy were immediately placed. Similar restrictions were also followed in other countries, including the UK. The study did, however, show evidence indicating benefit in preventing colorectal cancer and fractures.

2004—Initial Results of the Premarin® Division

The synthetic estrogen-only (Premarin®) trial was halted in February 2004, after an average follow-up of 6.8 years had shown a *slight* increased risk of stroke, without any cardiac benefits. The results also revealed a *decreased* risk of breast cancer and osteoporotic fractures. **The *decrease* in breast cancer risk in patients who received CEE alone was a differentiation from the CEE/ MPA treatment.**

The panic and mania resulting from the results of the CEE/MPA division overshadowed the positive results of CEE in reducing breast cancer.

Mishandling of results

The WHI study created unprecedented controversies, panic, and confusion. The chaos started in 2002, when the initial results from the combination (CEE/MPA) part of the study showed an increase in breast cancer and blood clots. The estrogen-only arm was halted due to a slight increase in strokes, yet it showed a decrease in breast cancer. The suspicion that estrogen causes breast cancer was already circulating—without significant proof.

It was clear that synthetic progesterone was the hormone causing the increase in breast cancer, not the synthetic estrogen. However, physicians and the public missed this critical finding. As a result, the false conclusion that estrogen was linked to breast cancer has been solidified in decades of misinformation.

The WHI Study Aftermath

Immediately after the researchers announced the initial results in 2002, panicked physicians took women off HRT for menopausal symptoms, recommending antidepressants as a preferred alternative. Physicians did not realize or question the apparent flaws in the study. The standard response was, "How can a study designed by 'elite' investigators, with 28,000 women participating, followed up in the forty top clinical centers in the country, and funded by the government (to the tune of $650 million) be flawed?"

As mentioned previously, estrogen wrongly got the blame for breast cancer; MPA (the synthetic progesterone) escaped any bad press, and women continued to receive wrong information.

Europeans were not hesitant to call out this study as unethical and senseless. Importantly, estrogen by mouth was first suspected of causing an increased risk for blood clots in the 1960s. The package inserts of all oral estrogen preparations revealed this risk, but this did not stop researchers from using oral estrogen in more investigations.

Because of the negative findings, the WHI study investigators recommended that hormone therapy not be prescribed for chronic disease prevention in postmenopausal women.

Further Analysis of the WHI Study Data

Follow-up of the WHI study continued for thirteen years. Reanalysis of the WHI trial showed that HRT in younger women (fifty to fifty-nine years) or within ten years of menopause showed a *beneficial* effect on the cardiovascular system, *reducing* coronary artery disease and deaths from all causes.[17, 18, 19, 20, 21, 22]

Critics later argued that most women in this study were greater than ten years past menopause. Older women subjected to the damaging effects of synthetic hormones are more vulnerable than younger women. This fact was and continues to be the main reason women older than age sixty or ten years past menopause seeking hormone replacement therapy encounter more significant resistance.

2005—Not Giving Up on Synthetic Hormones

By 2005, we still did not have sufficient clarity on estrogen's role on the cardiovascular system with all the studies done. It was not plausible to get the benefits of natural hormones in normal human doses (physiological doses) with *synthetic* hormones in low doses. Comparing synthetic and natural hormones is like comparing apples and oranges. They are both round fruit, but different in significant ways.

To recap, here's a summary of what we knew by 2005:

- The **Women's Health Initiative (WHI) study** showed that hormone replacement therapy was *ineffective* in preventing the new onset of cardiac events in previously healthy late menopausal women.

- The **Heart and Estrogen/Progestin Replacement Study (HERS)** failed to demonstrate *any benefit* of initiation of hormone therapy in women with established coronary heart disease.

Considering these results, researchers hypothesized that perhaps early initiation of hormone therapy in women who are just entering menopause would delay the onset of subclinical (early, undiagnosed) cardiovascular disease in women. Unfortunately, they did not consider using the correct hormones in the proper doses.

Kronos Early Estrogen Prevention Study (KEEPS)

KEEPS is the latest research to date. It began in 2005, shortly after the WHI study concluded in 2004.

KEEPS was a multicenter, five-year trial that studied women who had completed menopause within three years. Its purpose: to clarify our understanding of the effects of hormone replacement therapy on cardiovascular health, particularly preventing the progression of thickening of the carotid arteries in the neck, the accumulation of carotid calcium (plaques), and other health aspects.

Women between the ages of forty-two to fifty-eight received a:

1. Low dose conjugated equine estrogens (CEE) at the dose of 0.45 mg daily by mouth with twelve days of oral progesterone,

2. Weekly doses of 50 mcg transdermal (through the skin) estradiol, a bioidentical hormone, with twelve days of oral progesterone, or

3. Placebo.

Four-years results

Neither estrogen preparation with progesterone prevented the increase of carotid intimal medial thickness (plaques).

No adverse events, including venous thrombosis, were reported.

Topical (applied to the skin) estradiol improved sexual function.

Neither preparation affected cognition, breast pain, or skin wrinkling.

Researchers concluded the KEEPS, and its ancillary studies supported the use of hormone therapy.

KEEPS trial analysis

When we evaluate the KEEPS Trial, we note the pill of conjugated equine estrogen was a lower dose than that used in the WHI (0.45 mg for KEEPS versus 0.625 mg for WHI study). The dose was reduced to prevent blood clots, but it also contained an *insignificant* amount of estradiol; one that was too little to cause any benefits. Similarly, although identical to human estrogen, the estradiol's skin patch included *too low* a dose to provide any significant benefits once absorbed into the blood. Young, healthy women produce significantly more estradiol than was given in the skin patch.

Progesterone by mouth breaks down to many other steroids before reaching the blood, which further complicates trying to reproduce the benefits of a natural hormone environment. The KEEPS trial used bioidentical progesterone rather than medroxyprogesterone acetate (MPA). It was a significant advancement due to the results from the WHI study, when MPA was recognized as causing an *increased* risk of breast cancer.

Other Studies

Other similar but smaller studies took place in Europe, but none of them gained any significant press coverage or importance.

The Danish Osteoporosis Prevention Study (DOPS)

The Danes designed a randomized trial involving 1,006 women who were treated early in menopause with 17-beta estradiol (the same estrogen that a woman's ovaries make) and norethisterone (synthetic progesterone). The study reported significantly *decreased* risk of heart failure and myocardial infarction when hormone replacement therapy was started early in postmenopause.

The women who used estradiol alone had a significant reduction in breast cancer.[23]

Summary of the Studies

Uncontrolled studies (no control group or placebo and are weak studies):

- **Nurses' Health Study**

  Used self-reported data.
  Mainly used synthetic hormones.
  Participants had an increased breast cancer.
  There was a reduction in coronary artery disease.
  Increased stroke.

- **Million Women Study**

  Used self-reported data.
  Mainly used synthetic hormones.
  Participants had an increased breast cancer.

Controlled studies

- **HERS and HERS II**

  Used synthetic hormones.
  Postmenopausal HRT showed no cardiovascular benefit.
  No increase in breast cancer.

- **Women's Health Initiative Study**

  Used synthetic hormones.
  No breast cancer with synthetic estrogen.
  Increased breast cancer with synthetic progesterone.

- **KEEPS Study**

  Used low dose human estrogen (by mouth or transdermal).
  Used oral progesterone.
  No increase in breast cancer.

- **Danish Study**

  Used bioidentical estrogen and synthetic progesterone.
  No increase in breast cancer.
  Reduced heart failure and myocardial infarction (when started early).

Big Pharma's Influence

The pharmaceutical industry has heavily influenced the medical school curriculum for decades. Many physicians are still convinced that synthetic hormones are the same as bioidentical hormones. Most don't know the different estrogens produced by the human body because the medical curriculum does not teach about it. Until the pharmaceutical companies marketed the estrogen patch, most physicians ignored that oral estrogen causes blood clots (a well-known medical fact, due to the first pass effect of the liver).

The pharmaceutical industry not only heavily influences medical schools and the medical curriculum, but also has tremendous power over the government and its associated bodies.

Difficulty Being Heard, Especially Older Women

For decades, women seeking help for menopause symptoms were commonly shunned by doctors. Women more than ten years beyond menopause are still receiving resistance in getting bioidentical hormone replacement therapy from their physicians. This ten-year limit is a result of an erroneous conclusion from the WHI study "showing" that older women in the study had the most ill effects. As a result, women are taking prescription medications for insomnia, depression, and other menopausal symptoms. Many women seek therapies in alternative medicine and use all sorts of concoctions, including CBD (cannabidiol).

Bioidentical Hormones

Other than the UK, several European countries focused heavily on bioidentical hormones for at least the past two decades. These hormones are identical to what the human body makes.

Dr. John Lee and Dr. Johnathan Wright introduced bioidentical hormones in the US around the 1990s, but bioidentical hormones didn't gain popularity until the mid-2000s. Shortly afterward, some American physicians started to acknowledge the benefits of bioidentical hormones.

No research has been done only using bioidentical hormones administered to the skin and in physiological (normal human) ranges.

A Great Advancement in the UK

The US is using bioidentical hormones in various preparations and prescribing several other preparations of synthetic hormones. The UK recently made some progress, and the National Health Services (NHS) are prescribing low doses of "body-identical" (same as bioidentical but made by pharmaceutical companies) hormones for the relief of menopausal symptoms. However, they are not yet prescribing them for the purpose of preventing chronic diseases.

Current Recommendation in the US

Currently, in the US, hormone replacement therapy is recommended as an effective therapy for short-term treatment of menopausal symptoms and symptomatic, newly menopausal women who are age below sixty or within ten years of menopause.

Where We Are Today

Many women and physicians are aware of the safety and importance of bioidentical hormones. Women are becoming more comfortable pursuing therapy to treat menopausal symptoms and the prevention of age-related diseases.

The remnants of the Nurses' Health Study and the Million Women Study and their widely published results still lurk in the minds of most physicians. Most physicians have never looked at the studies but have instead relied on hearsay from their mentors and continue to pass inaccurate messages to their patients and colleagues.

Instruction in bioidentical hormone therapy is not part of the medical school curriculum. As a result, women continue to receive resistance from physicians who do not understand why hormones became controversial. Searching the literature and understanding the hormone controversy is a complex and arduous task. For physicians who do not comprehend this complex topic, the thought of "doing harm"—or anything that may lead to litigation—makes it easy to become dismissive.

Bioidentical hormone replacement therapy resolves menopausal symptoms, but much more importantly, when correctly dosed and administered, it dramatically slows down the diseases of aging. This has not reached mainstream medicine yet. But we are moving in the right direction, and there is hope.

Summary

- The benefits of estradiol were realized by the 1930s. As soon as estradiol was able to be extracted from the urine of pregnant women, a Canadian pharmaceutical company started to manufacture synthetic estrogen, which was made with the urine of pregnant horses. This synthetic estrogen was completely different from estradiol, the estrogen made by the human body.

- The Canadian pharmaceutical company merged with an American company to become Wyeth and dominated the market through their influence on the FDA and the medical institutions for over sixty years.

- No study was ever done using the hormones that a human body makes, in the doses the human body makes, nor administered in a safe way. All the major studies were conducted using synthetic (fake) hormones, trying to reproduce the effects of the bioidentical hormones made by the human body.

- Hormone use is controversial due to years of failed studies. Researchers were unable to replicate the results of bioidentical hormones with synthetic hormones. Synthetic hormones cause further harm when taken by mouth. Synthetic (or fake) progesterone is linked to breast cancer.

- Doctors have been kept in ignorance, not being taught that synthetic hormones are not the same as bioidentical, nor that by-mouth estrogen causes blood clots (topical estrogen does not). Also, physicians are not taught that fake progesterone is linked to breast cancer, while the progesterone that the human body makes is protective for the breast, reducing the risk of breast cancer.

- As a result, progress in the field of bioidentical hormone replacement therapy has been slow, but it is slowly moving in the right direction.

2

WHAT ARE HORMONES, AND WHY DO WE NEED THEM?

Hormones are potent chemicals (molecules) produced within our bodies. They control how the body works and affect a balanced, healthy life.

Our bodies make most hormones throughout life; the effects can be detrimental if they are out of normal ranges. For example, if insulin, thyroid hormone, or any of the adrenal gland hormones are out of balance, we need urgent medical attention.

Steroid hormones perform their functions by entering the cell, binding to the DNA, and initiating life-sustaining actions.

Every hormone naturally produced by the body has a unique structure and set of functions. The way that hormones interact with the body and each other is incredibly complex. At best, we only partially understand this magnificently intricate universe of hormones.

Although hormone replacement therapy for the symptoms of menopause has just recently been approved, hormone replacement therapy for the prevention of age-related diseases is not yet part of mainstream medicine. Big Pharma has complete influence over the government and the medical system, hindering medical advancement. Therefore, we should understand the basics, so that we can make an educated decision on how we decide to age.

This short chapter provides an understanding of the important facts related to hormones, and what we need to know about them. The basic concepts are simple and logical. You can make informed and educated choices when inundated with different opinions from different sources.

The body makes at least fifty different hormones. Hormone-producing cells make up specialized structures called glands, such as the ovaries, testes, thyroid gland, pancreas, and adrenal glands. Hormones can also be made in the cells of organs such as the brain, digestive tract, and liver.

Once produced, hormones can work in a locally controlled environment, such as the brain and the gut, or they can be released from glands into the bloodstream and travel to the rest of the body, where they can regulate the body's function.

All the different types of hormones in the body have specific signaling capabilities and exert influence on each other. This incredibly complex system, the endocrine system, allows proper body functioning.

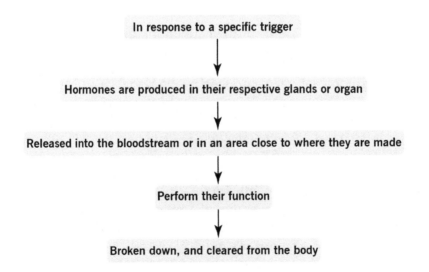

Diagram 2

Other than estradiol and progesterone in women, your body makes almost all other hormones throughout your life. Testosterone production in men starts to decline significantly after age fifty, but men do not abruptly stop producing it, unlike estradiol and progesterone. The decline in estradiol, progesterone, and testosterone affects the overall balance of other hormones in the body, which further contributes to the degenerative changes of aging.

Mitochondria and hormones

Mitochondria are tiny structures in cells where many critical, life-sustaining actions take place. Among the many fundamental roles of mitochondria are cellular energy production (without which there is no life) and regulation of oxidation stress that is due to the production of free radicals. Sex steroids (estradiol, progesterone, and testosterone) have important influences in energy production and management of the processes within the mitochondria of every cell in the body, especially in the cells of the nervous system and skeletal muscles, where cells have the highest activity.[24]

Examples of a Few Commonly Recognized Glands and Some of the Hormones They Make

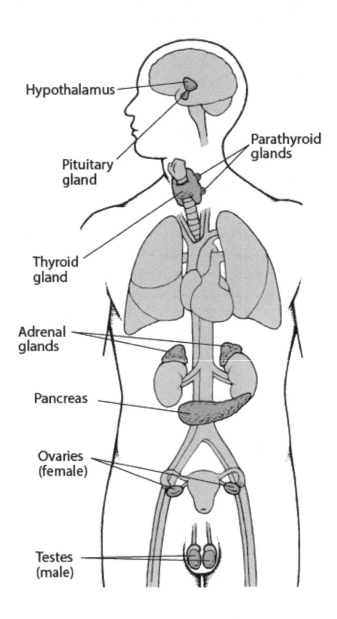

Diagram 3: Human body showing different glands.

Pancreas: The pancreas makes insulin. We cannot survive without insulin. Insufficient insulin production leads to diabetes. The pancreas also produces glucagon, which is critical for glucose balance, along with insulin.

Thyroid gland: Thyroid hormone is made in the thyroid gland. This is another commonly recognized hormone that is essential for life. The greater the imbalance in thyroid hormone levels, the greater the level of disease.

Adrenal gland: Adrenal glands are necessary for life, and our health depends on the balance of hormones that they produce. Cortisol and several other critically essential hormones are made in the adrenal glands.

Brain: The brain has glands and other specialized areas that produce vital hormones, which control the production and balance of hormones in different body parts.

Testes: Testes are male-specific glands and make testosterone. (See chapters 11 and 12 on testosterone.) Testosterone production spikes at puberty/adolescence and peaks in the late teens and early twenties. After age thirty, testosterone production drops by about one percent a year. Although men do not have a sharp decline in testosterone as women do with estradiol and progesterone, men usually reach a perceptibly low level of testosterone (andropause) in their early fifties.

Ovaries: Ovaries are female-specific glands and make estradiol and progesterone. (See chapters 5 and 6, respectively, on progesterone and estradiol.)

At menarche—the onset of the menstrual cycle—the ovaries make estradiol and progesterone in a specific cycle month after month. This cycle is naturally interrupted by pregnancy or unnaturally by birth control pills or hormonal imbalances.

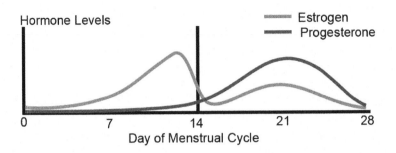

Diagram 4: The menstrual cycle.

Over time, the ovaries age, and both the quality and quantity of eggs deteriorates. During fetal life, there are several million eggs in the ovaries. This number reduces to about one million at birth, about 300,000 at puberty, and down to about 1,000 at menopause. In addition to the decrease of egg production, the production of hormones by the ovaries decreases as we age. From about forty to fifty years old, there is a significant reduction in estradiol and progesterone production, and women start having mild, intermittent symptoms of menopause. By an average age of fifty-one, the ovaries stop producing estradiol and progesterone, a state known as menopause.

Balance of Hormones

When most people are in their late twenties and thirties, hormone balance is typically at its best, as is their overall state of health.

All hormones have essential roles and work in communication with each other. We need a balance of all hormones for optimal health.

Significant imbalance or disruption in other hormones can affect ovulation and the production of estradiol and progesterone. Similarly, the loss of estradiol, progesterone, and other hormone systems negatively affects health.

Different patterns of hormone production

Hormones are produced in specific patterns and times. Some hormones, such as insulin and glucagon, for example, are made on-demand (to control blood glucose levels). Other hormones, such as cortisol, melatonin, and growth hormone, are made at specific times of the day. Melatonin and growth hormone are produced at night, when they can work on the repair and restorative functions.

Cortisol production spikes in the morning and is low at night, which helps us to sleep at night and be revitalized in the morning. Estradiol and progesterone production follows a unique monthly cycle. Certain brain hormones are made in pulsatile doses, and, if replaced in a continuous dose, do not work well.

Abnormal Hormone Levels

When most hormones are below normal, healthy ranges (physiological levels), it is considered a medical condition or disease and treated accordingly. For example, medical diseases arise when there is a lack of:

- insulin,
- thyroid hormone,
- cortisol,
- aldosterone,
- growth hormone (in children), or
- other brain-originating hormones.

Medical treatment usually involves addressing the hormone imbalance.

The decline in estradiol and progesterone in women and testosterone in men contributes to many diseases of aging. It is directly responsible for the loss of function and quality of life. The reduction in these hormones is considered "normal." However, the cycle of life, aging, and becoming senile is also "normal." The irony in medicine is that the medical and pharmaceutical systems make the most money from treating aging-related diseases. Healthcare providers do not dismiss osteoporotic fractures, coronary artery disease, hypertension, dyslipidemia (abnormal cholesterol levels), depression, and dementia, as might be expected, but rather provide costly medical treatment or surgery.

Over the decades after menopause, there is a gradual and continuous loss of health and well-being. Every part and function of the brain and body ages and deteriorates. The life expectancy for men and women who have healthy lifestyles and do not suffer from any major diseases is well into their nineties. Men and women live about four decades beyond andropause and menopause, respectively, when health and well-being continue to deteriorate. Most degeneration areas are in the musculoskeletal, brain, and nervous systems.

Although the body is designed to age and deteriorate after the decline of estradiol, progesterone (in women), and testosterone (in males), our DNA doesn't change. It can respond to the signals of these hormones once they are reintroduced.

Physiological (normal, healthy levels) hormone replacement for the prevention of age-related diseases has still not reached mainstream medicine. Until very recently, healthcare providers dismissed or treated the temporary symptoms of menopause with inappropriate medications, such as antidepressants and sleeping pills. Now, healthcare providers recently started treating symptoms of menopause with low dose hormones for a limited time.

By correctly replacing estradiol and progesterone in women and testosterone in men, we can live the decades beyond fifty with a much higher quality of life, well-being, and functionality.

Healthcare providers are not all knowledgeable about hormone replacement therapy because they do not receive a complete education about it in medical or nurse practitioner school or training. However, this information is very much part of the scientific and medical literature. Alternative medicine providers are not trained in hormone replacement therapy either and usually focus on non-medical therapies with little scientific basis.

3

BIOIDENTICAL AND SYNTHETIC HORMONES—BIOCHEMISTRY MADE EASY

This chapter highlights some simple, basic biochemistry knowledge about hormones and hormone replacement, so that we can appreciate the critical difference between similar-looking hormones—specifically, bioidentical hormones versus synthetic hormones—which have profoundly different effects on our body.

Atoms

Atoms are the **smallest unit of matter** that have unique chemical characteristics. Commonly recognized atoms are hydrogen, oxygen, sodium, chloride, magnesium, carbon, and sulfur, with the hydrogen atom being the smallest atom. The periodic table identifies all the atoms discovered to date.

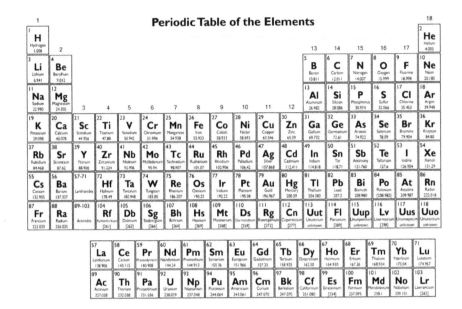

Diagram 5: The periodic table.

Molecule

Molecules are unique substances created from a specific combination and sequence of atoms and are the **smallest fundamental unit of a chemical compound**.

Molecules have a three-dimensional structure with a unique shape, atomic environment, and character.

Common simple molecules that we recognize are:

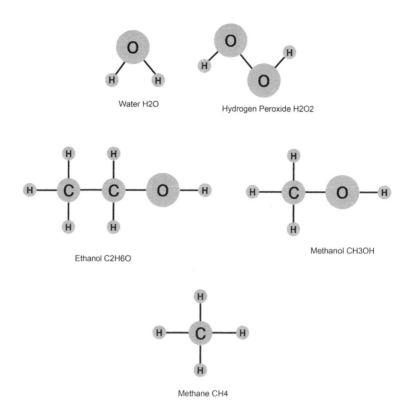

Diagram 6

1. Water: H_2O, made from two hydrogen atoms and one oxygen.

2. Hydrogen peroxide: H_2O_2, made from two hydrogen atoms and two oxygen atoms.

3. Ethanol: $CH_3\text{-}CH_2\text{-}OH$, made from two carbon atoms, six hydrogen atoms, and one oxygen atom.

4. Methanol: $CH_3\text{-}OH$, made from one carbon atom, four hydrogen atoms, and one oxygen atom.

5. Methane: CH_4, made from one carbon and four hydrogen atoms.

Hormones are also molecules, built from atoms in a specific sequence. A few examples are:

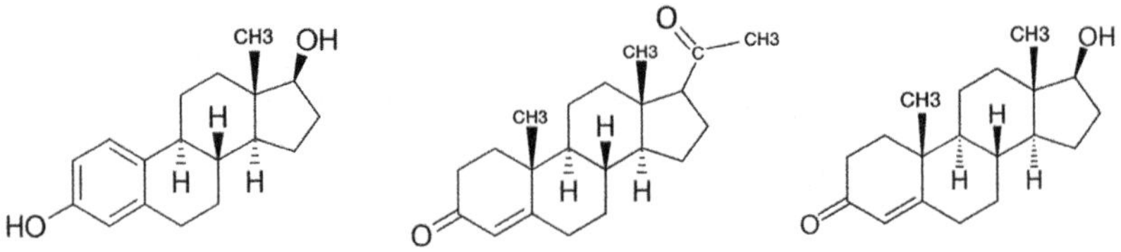

Estradiol   Progesterone   Testosterone

Diagram 7

1. Estradiol,
2. Progesterone, and
3. Testosterone.

Atoms and molecules are unique. Think of how letters make up a word. Atoms combine in a specific sequence to construct a molecule similar to how letters combine to construct a word. Adding, removing, or changing the sequence of an atom will create a different molecule, the same way that adding, removing, or changing the sequence of letters will change the meaning of a word.

Molecules work with other molecules and DNA. As mentioned previously, the 3-D arrangement of atoms creates a molecule, which has a unique shape and properties. Adding, removing, or changing the 3-D structure of atoms will change the shape and character of the molecule. Some similarities may remain, but there will be a lot of differences too.

The Cell

A cell is the smallest functional unit of an organism. It is a closed structure where the work of living takes place. Molecules go in and out of the cells through special receptors (doors).

Hormones are molecules that act as messengers, telling the cell's DNA what to make so that the body can function correctly. Some molecules, such as certain steroid hormones, can enter cells with and without receptors.

The cell is a highly complex structure that contains thousands of crucial, intricate, life-sustaining structures, including mitochondria and DNA. Different organs have different types of cells, but the DNA in every cell is the same.

A cell's DNA is in a separate protected compartment within the cell, the nucleus. Hormones enter the cell, then the nucleus, and then attach to specific areas of DNA, triggering the production of life-sustaining and body-regulating substances. This process of entering the cell, then the nucleus, and attaching to DNA is highly complex and has multiple checkpoints. Hormones are messenger molecules with unique properties and structures; substituting hormones with a different hormone will mean that the process will not work the same way.

Enzymes

Enzymes are molecules that break down other molecules and substances. One of the many vital functions of enzymes is to change one molecule to another, by altering the molecule's atoms, creating a different molecule. Enzymes are extremely specific in their function. They also have a unique, three-dimensional shape, which fits specifically into the target molecules so that it can be effectively altered or broken down.

Most enzymes are made in the liver, pancreas, and digestive tract.

Healthcare providers do not recommend patients swallow hormones. Hormones would have a long trip: enter the stomach, go through the digestive tract, pass through the liver, and get into the blood. In the process, the hormones would encounter many enzymes and pH changes and trigger undesired reactions in the liver. As noted in chapter 5, "Progesterone," if a person swallowed progesterone, much of it would be metabolized into other steroids. This conversion is inconsistent and depends on many internal factors that we neither understand well nor can predictably control.

Bioidentical and Synthetic Hormones

Bioidentical

When you encounter the term *bioidentical*, note it is an arbitrary term relating to hormones, meaning that the molecular structure of a hormone is completely identical to what the human body makes.

One of the most common questions asked about bioidentical hormones is, "Where do they come from?" It is important to understand, regardless of their source, that the main concern should be if the product is of the highest grade and purity, and meets USP standards. USP stands for US Pharmacopeia, and it sets the bar for potency and purity of chemicals to meet pharmaceutical grade, which is the highest grade for a chemical.

Is the estradiol or progesterone that is being compounded purified to the highest level under USP guidelines? The estradiol and progesterone prepared by compounding pharmacies meets USP standards. Estradiol is extracted and purified from soy. Progesterone is extracted and purified from yams.

See Diagram 8 for examples of bioidentical estrogens: These are called bioidentical because they are made by the human body.

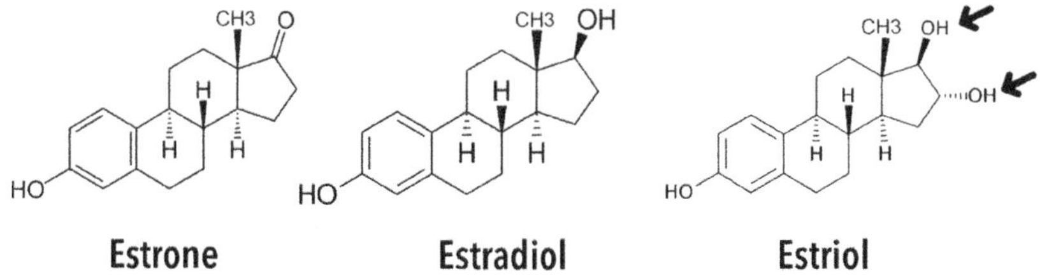

Estrone   **Estradiol**   **Estriol**

Diagram 8: Bioidentical estrogens.

The human body makes progesterone, which has critical and specific functions, including protection for the breast and brain. Synthetic versions of progesterone are molecularly altered, and not only do they not provide all the benefits of bioidentical progesterone, they have also been linked to breast cancer.

Synthetic

When referring to hormones, synthetic means that the molecule made by the body has been molecularly altered with a changed sequence, arrangement, or number of atoms. It is not the same product anymore. The synthetic version may retain some of the properties of the original molecule, but it is a unique molecule whose only known advantage is that pharmaceutical companies can patent it.

Premarin®, also known as conjugated equine estrogens (CEE), is a mixture of several estrogens derived from the urine of pregnant horses, and those are very different from the estrogens made by the human body. In fact, it is because of this degree of difference that Premarin® (CEE) is patentable.

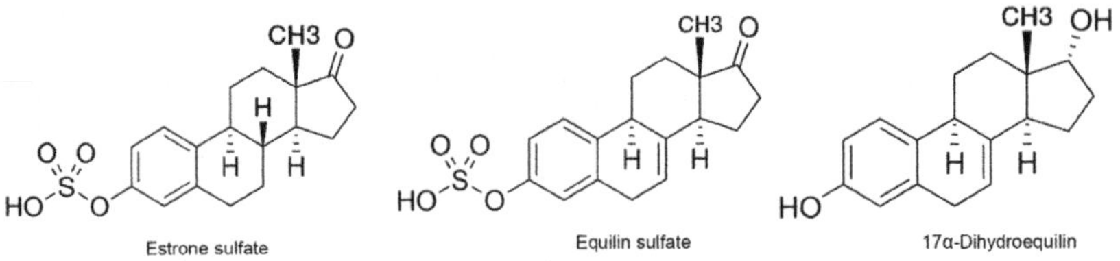

Estrone sulfate   Equilin sulfate   17α-Dihydroequilin

Diagram 9: Synthetic estrogens.

Medroxyprogesterone acetate (MPA) has been the most widely used synthetic progesterone. MPA is created in a lab. The only known feature that it shares with real (bioidentical) progesterone is that it causes the uterine lining to shed after building up by estradiol. This was the synthetic progesterone used in the Women's Health Initiative study, and it caused an increase in breast cancer.

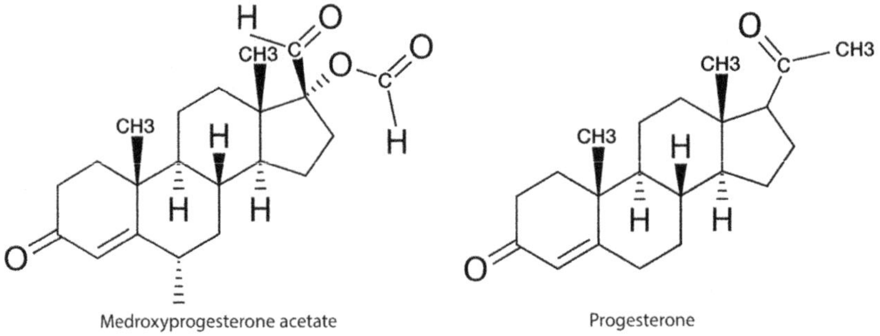

Medroxyprogesterone acetate   Progesterone

Diagram 10: MPA and bioidentical progesterone.

Molecular Integrity

Rearranging, removing, or adding atoms to a molecule will change its properties. Some similarities may remain, but there will undoubtedly be differences and potentially harmful properties.

For example, ethanol and methanol are two different types of alcohol. Ethanol is the alcohol used in beverages and certain medications; it is relatively safe to ingest. Methanol has many industrial uses, including fuel and construction materials. The molecular difference between ethanol and methanol is CH_2, which is one carbon atom and two hydrogen atoms. If mixed in an alcoholic beverage, they taste similar and cause similar effects, but methanol is poisonous and causes blindness.

Molecular integrity is critically important to hormones. As in the example of ethanol versus methanol, hormones that have similar-sounding names, similar (but not identical) atoms and atomic arrangements can still cause widely different reactions, especially in the long run. Many physicians are still under the influence of Big Pharma and believe that bioidentical and synthetic hormones are the same.

Healthcare providers who prescribe replacement hormones should select a bioidentical hormone. Our cells, DNA, and enzymes function correctly with bioidentical hormones. It makes no sense to use altered (synthetic) versions of a hormone to perform the function of a bioidentical hormone.

4

ESTROGEN

Estrogen is a powerful steroid hormone that physically interacts with DNA to initiate essential functions of the body. There are many different estrogen-like molecules in nature made by plants and animals.

A human female only makes three specific types of estrogen: estradiol, estrone, and estriol. Each estrogen differs slightly in molecular structure but has quite different functions on the cell's DNA.

Estradiol

Estradiol is the most critical and potent estrogen. At normal (physiological) levels and balanced with progesterone, it allows women to function in optimum health. Normal, healthy estradiol levels need to be balanced with normal progesterone ranges. When estradiol is *not* produced in normal ranges, the body will start to deteriorate, which happens after menopause.

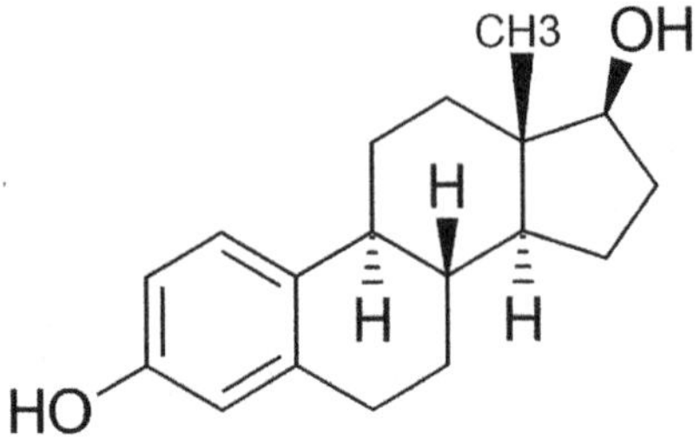

Estradiol

Diagram 11

Since the 1940s, pharmaceutical companies (Big Pharma) have viewed estradiol as a threat, because it cannot be patented. This resulted in ongoing attempts to label it harmful, making way for molecularly altered versions that can be patented. After many decades of reading Big Pharma's false claims, mainstream healthcare providers have realized that estradiol is the only estrogen that a woman should receive when replacement is needed. Pharmaceutical companies recently started producing medications containing more natural estradiol products than synthetic versions.

The ovaries produce more than 90 percent of the estradiol in a woman's body. The rest is made from converting androgens, such as testosterone, from the adrenal glands by enzymes (aromatase) made by the liver.

Men also produce a small amount of estradiol, converted from the testosterone, produced by the testes or adrenal glands.

Functions of estradiol

Estradiol affects every function of the body. Along with progesterone, it has numerous effects on the functioning and balance of the body. Also, estradiol optimizes the effects of other hormones.

Estradiol promotes the biosynthesis of complex molecules and structures, such as bone, different types of muscle, skin, the brain, the nervous system, and so much more. (Chapters 6 through 10 describe these benefits.)

The absence of estradiol and progesterone marks the onset of rapid aging. Hot flashes and night sweats are the only temporary symptoms of menopause. Other symptoms, such as foggy brain, loss of libido, vaginal dryness, low energy, poor sleep, weight gain and difficulty losing weight, and body composition changes may stabilize with time; but they don't all go away, and women adjust to them.

Estriol

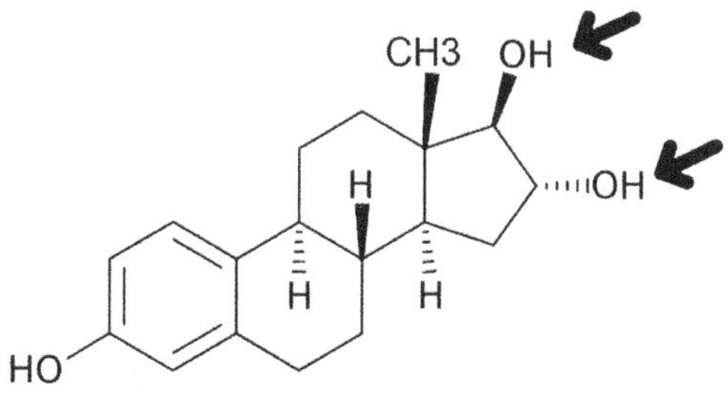

Estriol

Diagram 12

Estriol is a metabolic product of estradiol. After estradiol is produced in the ovaries and released into the blood, some of it converts to estriol in the urogenital area. Estriol has no known effects in places other than the genital and urological system.

Estriol allows vaginal lubrication and helps maintain healthy structures of the vaginal and urological system. The body produces an incredibly high amount of estriol during pregnancy, facilitating changes in the birth canal in preparation for delivery. Adequate production or supplementation of estradiol will internally convert to sufficient estriol levels.

In non-pregnant women, estriol is produced only as an irreversible metabolite (byproduct) of estradiol. Due to the importance of estriol in maintaining healthy tissue in the genital and urological system, many physicians prescribe estriol for vaginal dryness and thinning. If estradiol is in normal (physiological) ranges, enough will convert to estriol, and vaginal dryness will resolve. If there is vaginal dryness present, the body's estradiol levels are undoubtedly low.

Estrone

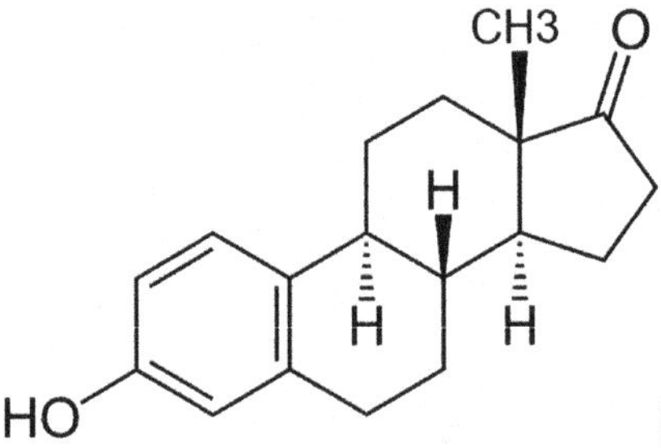

Estrone

Diagram 13

As the weakest form of estrogen, **estrone** is the predominate form of estrogen remaining after menopause. The ovaries make a small amount; the rest is converted from androgens (testosterone, androstenedione, DHEA) in places such as fat cells. Estrone can reversibly convert to estradiol as well as directly and irreversibly convert to estriol. It is the storage form of estrogen.

Replacing Estrogen

Triest

In the early days of bioidentical hormone replacement therapy, anti-aging physicians prescribed Triest—short for Tri-estrogen, a combination of the three human estrogens—estradiol, estrone, and estriol. The physicians reasoned that these are the naturally occurring estrogens in the human body. After a while, they feared estrone might have inflammatory properties without providing any benefits. As a consequence, anti-aging physicians prescribed Biest.

Biest

Biest is the combination of estriol and estradiol. For many years, Biest was the estrogen preparation of choice. Due to a lack of understanding of the importance and functions of estradiol and the false belief that estradiol is linked to breast cancer, this combination was more popular than giving estradiol alone.

Estradiol is the only estrogen that should be given for replacement. The active hormone allows the body to perform at its best when in normal doses and correctly balanced with progesterone.

5

PROGESTERONE

Progestogens are a class of hormones. The name ***progesterone*** refers only to the body's natural hormones. Fake or synthetic versions of progesterone are called similar, but *misleading* words such as **progestin**.

At one time, scientists believed that progesterone's *primary* function was to regulate the inner lining of the uterus. Unfortunately, many physicians still believe this. Progesterone has many other indispensable roles in the body.

Production of Progesterone

Fertile women make progesterone in the ovaries for about two weeks every month in the second part of the menstrual cycle. During pregnancy, the uterus and placenta make a lot more progesterone. By the third trimester, the body produces about ten times more progesterone than the peak production during the menstrual cycle.

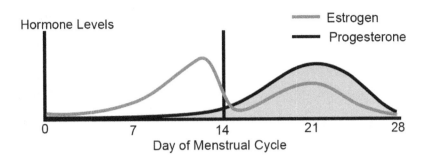

Diagram 14: Progesterone phase of the menstrual cycle.

The adrenal glands and the brain of both men and women make a small amount of progesterone.

How the Body Produces Progesterone

Progesterone is a steroid hormone, as are estradiol, testosterone, DHEA, cortisol, and aldosterone, among others. Cholesterol is the origin of all steroid hormones. Once cholesterol enters the cell, it is metabolized to different steroid hormones, depending on various factors.

Pregnenolone is the first steroid hormone made from cholesterol. Pregnenolone directly converts to progesterone. After going through a chain of reactions facilitated by specific enzymes and under particular internal environments, progesterone will convert to other hormones, including cortisol, aldosterone, estrone, estradiol, and testosterone.

If a person swallowed progesterone, much of it would be metabolized into other steroids. This conversion is inconsistent and depends on many internal factors that we don't understand well or control. This inconsistent conversion is the main reason that we avoid taking progesterone by mouth.

Progesterone Effects on the Body

Progesterone has numerous direct functions as well as the task of balancing the effects of estradiol. (See chapter 4 for an explanation of estradiol.)

Progesterone, Breast, and Uterine Tissue

Progesterone has critically important effects on maintaining healthy breast tissue. Women who do not make enough progesterone during their menstrual cycle often have various breast problems, such as breast cysts and uterine fibroids.

Whereas bioidentical progesterone helps to protect the breast from cancer, *synthetic* progesterone is the only hormone linked to breast cancer.

Progesterone and Mood

Progesterone maintains countless essential functions of the brain, the nervous system, and psychological well-being. It is necessary for balancing mood and eliminating anxiety. *Synthetic* progesterone does not produce the calming effects of natural progesterone. (See chapter 6 for more details on progesterone effects on the brain.)

In menstruating women, estradiol that is not balanced by progesterone results in PMS (premenstrual syndrome) and PMDD (premenstrual dysphoric disorder).

Progesterone and Pregnancy

Without normal levels of progesterone, pregnancy can't take place. Although synthetic progesterone can trigger sloughing of the inner lining of the uterus and cause menstrual bleeding, there is no substitute for bioidentical progesterone for preparing the uterus lining for pregnancy or maintaining pregnancy.

Cardiovascular Effects

Progesterone has beneficial effects on the cardiovascular system, including blood vessel walls. It reduces blood pressure by relaxing blood vessel walls. In addition, it has similar effects to certain blood pressure-lowering medications (calcium channel blockers) and has diuretic properties (stimulating urination) through its impact on the kidneys.

In contrast, progestins (synthetic progesterone) have blood pressure-increasing effects and are responsible for creating a state that leads to blood clot formation.[25]

Respiratory System

Improved lung function can be linked to progesterone, due to the hormone's powerful anti-inflammatory properties. During the COVID-19 pandemic, a clinical trial at Cedar Sinai Medical Center, Los Angeles, showed that progesterone injection (100 mg twice daily) improved outcomes in hypoxemic (low oxygen saturation) men with moderate to severe COVID-19.[26]

6

ESTRADIOL AND PROGESTERONE
EFFECTS ON THE BRAIN

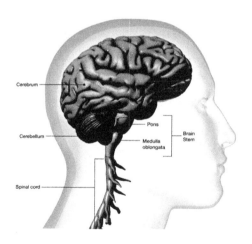

Diagram 15

This chapter describes some of the many critical ways that estrogen and progesterone profoundly affect the brain and nervous system.

The nervous system controls every function of the body by transmitting signals from the brain to the end target, such as the internal organs, glands, and various other structures.

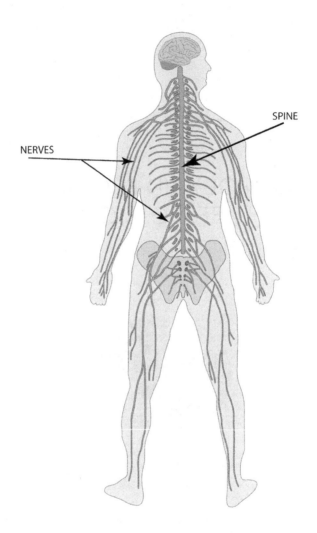

Diagram 16: Brain, spinal cord, and nerves.

As the center of the nervous system, the brain is composed of approximately *100 billion* neurons (brain cells) and *billions* of other types of cells that support the neurons. The brain extends to the spinal cord, from which nerves branch off to every part of the body. The neuron's supporting cells, numerous brain chemicals (neurotransmitters), and brain-originating hormones form an extremely complex system.

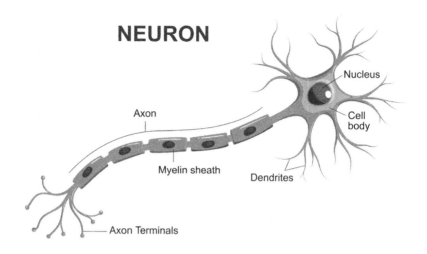

Diagram 17

Declining levels of estradiol and progesterone as part of the aging process cause the progressive degeneration of the brain and nervous system. This decline results in advancing age-related neurodegenerative diseases, senile dementia, slowed response time, a decrease in balance, and so much more.

Higher brain functions, such as memory, cognition, learning, fine motor skills, balance, emotions, mood, and motivation rely on normal (physiological) human ranges of estradiol and progesterone. Our brain functioning suffers from declining levels of estradiol and progesterone.

The Brain and Estrogen

During pregnancy, the remarkable effects of estradiol start to affect the fetus' developing brain and continue throughout life. Estradiol and estadiol receptors are at the highest levels in the brain both prenatally and during the first days of life, then gradually decline to adult levels.[27]

Estradiol has countless crucial roles in various neurological functions, including involvement in fine motor control, sensitivity to pain, emotions, mood, cognitive function, learning, memory, motor coordination, and strategies used to maintain balance.

Estrogen has anti-inflammatory and antioxidant properties that protect the brain against stroke damage and other neurological injuries. It helps to prevent neuropsychiatric disorders, such as Alzheimer's disease.

Effects of estrogen are so critical to health that studies suggest the brain can make estradiol directly from cholesterol.[28, 29] Additionally, men will convert testosterone to estradiol using a critical enzyme (P450) that is produced by the liver.

Estrogen and Cognitive Function

It is common for women to have apathy, memory loss, and a decrease in cognition after menopause.[30] Numerous research studies confirm estradiol's impact on cognitive function and psychological well-being.[31]

Estrogen affects the serotonergic, dopaminergic, noradrenergic, and anticholinergic systems.

Older adults are often troubled by memory loss. Estrogen helps to tackle this problem as it improves verbal memory. A well-designed study (*randomized, double-blind, placebo-controlled, crossover trial*) from 1996 through 1998 showed that estrogen in a therapeutic dose alters brain activation patterns in postmenopausal women by affecting specific brain regions during the performance of routine memory functions. The study used brain activation patterns measured during MRI imaging while the women performed tasks involving verbal and nonverbal working memory.[32]

Estrogen and Alzheimer's Dementia

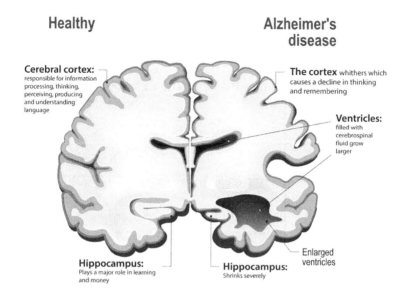

Healthy

Alzheimer's disease

Cerebral cortex: responsible for information processing, thinking, perceiving, producing and understanding language

The cortex whithers which causes a decline in thinking and remembering

Ventricles: filled with cerebrospinal fluid grow larger

Hippocampus: Plays a major role in learning and money

Hippocampus: Shrinks severely

Enlarged ventricles

Diagram 18: Normal brain vs. Alzheimer's brain.

Alzheimer's dementia is responsible for much disruption in the ability to care for oneself, leading to family, social, and economic costs. How can we prevent this terrible disease? Part of the answer is using estradiol, which acts as an antioxidant to reduce the nerve cell generation of beta amyloid. (Beta amyloid is a protein that forms in clumps in the brains of people with Alzheimer's disease. Scientists abbreviate beta as β.) Multiple studies indicate that postmenopausal estrogen replacement therapy may prevent or delay the onset of Alzheimer's dementia.[33, 34, 35]

Medication trials of estrogen therapy in women showed improved cognitive function in women who do not have dementia. In older women who take postmenopausal estrogen replacement therapy, there was a low incidence of death caused by Alzheimer's disease compared to those who did not take estrogen replacement therapy.

A twelve-year, population-based study in Cache County, Utah, examined the association between estrogen and cognitive decline in over 2,000 older adults. The study showed two critical factors associated with better-performing brain function later in life:

1. Hormone therapy use, and

2. The length of time that a woman's body produces endogenous estrogen. (The longer time enhances cognitive abilities.)[36]

Another study showed that women taking estrogen therapy had a milder form of Alzheimer's disease than those not taking it. Researchers concluded that administration of a closer to physiological (normal, human ranges) dose of estradiol enhances the memory and attention of postmenopausal women with Alzheimer's dementia.

Memory

Estrogen has powerful and profound effects on memory. One of women's most common complaints during perimenopause and menopause is "foggy brain." As women approach menopause, their ability to remember tasks and to multi-task declines. Over the years, women get used to the decrease in memory and may progress to senile dementia slowly.

Estrogen replacement therapy preserves cognitive function, protects against age-related memory decline, and decreases the risk for Alzheimer's disease in postmenopausal women.

Loss of estrogen after removal of ovaries impacts memory. Studies done on women who underwent hysterectomies with the removal of their ovaries confirm this conclusion. Memory tests completed before and after treating with estrogen versus placebo (an inactive substance that has no medication) demonstrated the profound effect of estrogen on memory.[37]

Other studies, where women underwent hysterectomy with intact ovaries and circulating estrogen, showed stable cognitive function.[38]

Long-term use of estrogen replacement therapy provides many benefits. A proton MR spectroscopy study compared women who had been using long-term estrogen replacement therapy versus nonusers (women who did not take estrogen replacement therapy). Nonusers had a higher concentration of choline-containing compounds, which negatively affect nerve cells.[39]

> **Choline-containing compounds were much higher in non-estrogen replacement therapy users than in estrogen replacement therapy users and young women. Choline-containing compounds are damaging and increase the rate at which cells break down.[39]**

Estrogen Effects on Pain

Estrogen helps in the pain pathways. Therefore, women are susceptible to pain at certain times in the menstrual cycle when estrogen levels are low. Studies concluded that the brain's natural painkiller system responds more powerfully to pain when estrogen levels are high.[40, 41]

Estrogen and Neuroprotection

Estradiol, directly and indirectly, stimulates nerve cell growth, is involved in nerve cell survival, and protects against neurotoxins that increase free radical production. (Free radicals are unstable atoms that can damage cells, causing illness and symptoms of aging, such as wrinkles, central nervous system and cardiovascular disease, and a host of other age-related changes.)

The brain depends on blood as a source of energy; one-third of the brain consists of blood vessels. Estrogen increases cerebral perfusion (blood flow) by binding to endothelial receptors (lining of blood vessels) and stimulating nitric oxide release, which leads to vasodilation (widened blood vessels), allowing better blood flow to the brain.

Estrogen protects nerve cells against damage caused by ischemic strokes (those caused by loss of blood flow). By increasing blood flow to the brain, estrogen provides anti-inflammatory effects, promotes neuronal synaptic activity, and provides neuroprotective and neurotrophic (nutritional) effects on the brain.[42, 43]

A study compared two-year longitudinal changes in regional cerebral blood flow. (The researchers measured changes that occurred at intervals over two years.) It is possible to see the actual changes in blood flow associated with estrogen use. The two groups of women included those who used estrogen replacement therapy and those who did not. The women performed several memory tasks while researchers performed PET scan imaging of regional cerebral blood flow. Across a series of standardized neuropsychological tests of memory, estrogen users got higher scores than nonusers of comparable intellect.[44]

Estrogen interacts with neuroprotective intracellular signaling pathways and behaves as a neuroprotective antioxidant.[45] (Antioxidants lessen or prevent the harmful effects of free radicals by making the unstable atom more stable.)

Estrogen promotes the growth and repair of neurons and stimulates the production of nerve growth factors. Estrogen increases the level of serotonin, dopamine, and norepinephrine. It has neuroprotective effects against oxidative stress, ischemic (reduced blood flow) changes, and the damage caused by the β- amyloid protein that is involved in Alzheimer's disease.

The hippocampus is a part of the brain that is involved with learning and memory. Studies show that women who used estrogen therapy had larger left and right hippocampal sizes than men as well as larger right hippocampal volumes compared to past users and never-users of estrogen therapy.[46]

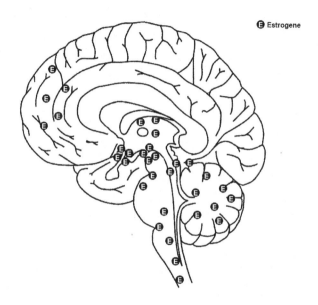

Diagram 19: Areas of high estradiol activity.

Estrogen and Depression

Estradiol helps with depression in both premenopausal and menopausal women. There have been numerous studies confirming this. A study published in the *Archives of General Psychiatry* in 2001 focused on premenopausal women with irregular periods who met the criteria for major depressive order, dysthymic disorder (mild, long-lasting depression), or minor depression. The women showed improvement in depression with transdermal estrogen (skin patches).[47]

Women with menopause and early postmenopause symptoms are at a two- to fourfold increased risk for clinically significant depressive symptoms. A well-designed (double-blind, placebo-controlled randomized) trial was done at the University of North Carolina at Chapel Hill from October 2010 to February 2016. Participants included euthymic women (in stable mental health) aged forty-five to sixty who were perimenopausal and early postmenopausal. The study reported that twelve months of transdermal estradiol plus intermittent micronized progesterone (a preparation broken down into very small particles) were more effective than a placebo in preventing the development of significant depressive symptoms.[48]

Progesterone and the Brain

What does progesterone do to enhance health? So far, we explored the many benefits of estrogen. Progesterone complements the effects of estrogen on the brain and has multiple essential functions in the nervous system.

Progesterone regulates mood, cognition, inflammation, mitochondrial function, neurogenesis and regeneration, nerve myelination, and recovery from traumatic brain injury.

The human ovaries produce progesterone for about two weeks in a month. Studies show that the ovarian progesterone production (intermittent) pattern has more significant benefits than continuous dosing.

Receptors for progesterone are on every type of nerve cell and throughout the brain, indicating progesterone's broad range of function in the nervous system.[49] Progesterone and its metabolites (the other hormones that it breaks down into) also help regulate other neurotransmitter systems.

Researchers who identified progesterone receptors in a specific brain area concluded that progesterone has vital functions in that area.

Some of the Areas of the Brain Shown to Have Abundant Progesterone Receptors

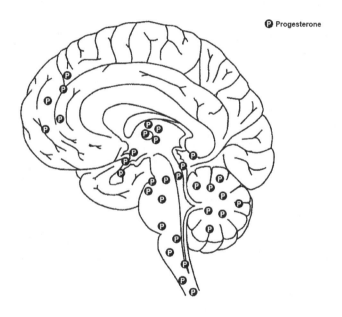

Diagram 20: Areas of high progesterone activity.

Thalamus: This area of the brain receives stimuli from the rest of the body, filters it, and then passes the stimuli to higher brain levels for processing. The thalamus also has a role in emotion, memory, arousal, and other associated functions.

Amygdala: Regulates emotion and memories, especially emotional memories.

Hippocampus: Area of the brain involved in learning and memory.

Hypothalamus: The hypothalamus has many functions. It releases other hormones, controls daily physiological cycles (such as sleeping and waking), controls appetite, manages sexual behavior, regulates emotional responses, regulates body temperature, and more.

Frontal cortex: This is the front part of the brain under the forehead. It is responsible for higher cognitive functions such as:

- memory,
- problem-solving,
- impulse control,
- social interactions,
- emotions,
- motor function (movement),
- decision-making,
- planning appropriate behavioral responses to external and internal stimuli, and
- attention, among many other functions.

Cognitive Effects of Progesterone

Estrogen upregulates (increases the number of) progesterone receptors in the brain. Studies show improved cognitive effects with estrogen and progesterone. A study measuring verbal testing and brain imaging with progesterone verified improved performance. The same results did *not* occur in women who took *synthetic* progesterone.[50]

Depression and Anxiety—Calming Effects of Progesterone

Progesterone helps prevent depression and anxiety by interacting with GABA, a potent neurotransmitter with calming effects on the mood. When progesterone breaks down to allopregnanolone, this increases GABA activity. Through this mechanism, progesterone produces a calming effect and eases anxiety.

Low levels of progesterone decrease serotonin, which can result in poor sleep and depression. Low progesterone levels cannot balance the stimulating effects of estrogen, which can, in turn, lead to anxiety.

Perimenopause is associated with a vulnerability to developing a depressive illness. Several studies confirmed an increased rate of new-onset major depressive episodes during the months surrounding menopause.[51] Women with no prior history of depression may become depressed during menopause.[52] And women who go into early menopause have an increased risk of severe depression.

Progesterone and its metabolites influence emotional processing. Medical professionals assert that these are critical for alleviating mood symptoms experienced by women with PMS (premenstrual syndrome) and PMDD (premenstrual dysphoric disorder; similar to premenstrual syndrome, but more serious). Women taking synthetic progesterone do not receive these benefits.

Progesterone and Traumatic Brain Injury

Research conducted over thirty years revealed a tremendous amount about the mechanisms behind traumatic brain injury. After traumatic brain injury, there is a release of many proinflammatory substances (cytokines) and oxidative stress reactions, which cause swelling and damage to the local brain, resulting in secondary brain injury.[53] (Oxidative stress is an imbalance between free radicals and antioxidants in the body.)

Progesterone suppresses many of the damaging reactions that result in secondary brain injury. As a result of the many protective effects of progesterone, cerebral edema (swelling) reduces, and more people survive in the critical hours following the trauma.

In addition to the ovaries and placenta, both women's and men's adrenal glands and brains provide progesterone. It is made from cholesterol in the brain by cells called oligodendrocytes and glial cells. Progesterone has a critical role in the balance and stability of the nervous system.[54] Studies over the last twenty years verified that progesterone has potent neuroprotective properties and maintains cellular health and survival.

Traumatic brain injury is complicated by a cascade of toxic events throughout the brain and body.[55]

There is evidence that progesterone plays a part in correcting and maintaining homeostasis after physiological stress and injury beyond the central nervous system.

Progesterone limits neuronal apoptosis (self-destruction) through inhibition of mitochondrial-specific proapoptotic enzymes. It maintains cellular integrity and survival by promoting mitochondrial regulation and stabilization. By similar mechanisms, progesterone infusion after traumatic brain injury limits the inflammatory response in other tissues and organs, including the spleen and gut.[56]

Two independent trials showed promising results for progesterone use after acute traumatic brain injury.

The progesterone for traumatic brain injury, experimental clinical trial III (ProTECT III) was a double-blinded study that randomized 100 patients with moderate to severe brain injury. Participants received either progesterone or placebo infusion within eleven hours of their traumatic event. Patients in the progesterone group showed a 50 percent reduction in thirty-day mortality compared with the controls. There were no serious adverse effects attributed to progesterone exposure.[57]

Another similar randomized, double-blinded, placebo-controlled study on 149 severely brain-injured patients (with a Glasgow Coma Score of less than eight, with fifteen being the highest possible score) showed mortality at six months to be 18 percent in the progesterone group. (Only 18 percent of those treated with progesterone died compared to 32 percent in the placebo group.) The progesterone group also demonstrated significantly higher favorable outcomes at three months and six-month intervals.[58]

Myelin Sheath Protection

The axon is a part of the nerve cell involved in the rapid transmission of information and is covered with a protective sheath made from a material called myelin. Progesterone is involved in the repair and synthesis of myelin proteins.[59]

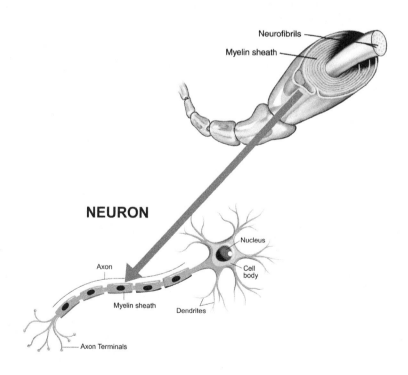

Diagram 21: Myelin sheath.

Summary

- Estradiol and progesterone have profound functional and protective effects on the brain.

- Every cell of the brain and nervous system requires estradiol and progesterone for optimal function.

- In men, a portion of testosterone is always converted to estradiol for the important benefits of estradiol.

- Age-related, senile dementia, and other age-related neurological diseases are significantly reduced with replacement of physiological levels of estradiol and progesterone.

- The "normal," expected decline in cognition, memory, and mental function with aging can be significantly prevented with correctly implemented hormone replacement.

- Age-related depression, anxiety, and other mood issues are largely resolved with proper hormone replacement therapy.

7

OSTEOPOROSIS AND OSTEOARTHRITIS

Our bones, muscles, ligaments, tendons, and cartilage keep us mobile, flexible, strong, and functional. But the combination of degenerative changes in these structures creates physical debility, joint pain, stiffness, and weakness with aging.

Osteoporosis

The term *osteoporosis* means "porous bone" and represents one of the most debilitating diseases of aging. It involves ongoing degeneration of the skeleton, resulting in progressive debility over the decades, causing a profound loss in quality of life. The consequences of osteoporosis and dementia are the two top reasons for losing independence, resulting in long-term nursing home placement.

Bone is a highly complex, metabolically active tissue made up of collagen proteins and mineralized substances, giving it properties of incredible strength and resistance.

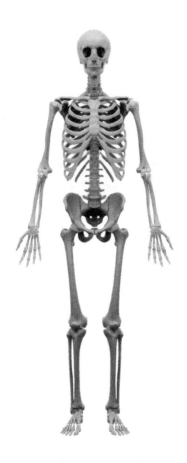

Diagram 22: Human skeleton.

The major functions of bone are:[60]

- Mechanical support.
- Protection of vital organs (e.g., brain and spinal cord, lungs, heart).
- Production of blood cells (in the bone marrow).
- Reservoir for essential minerals (calcium, phosphorous, etc.), growth factors, and osteocalcin (a small protein hormone).[61]

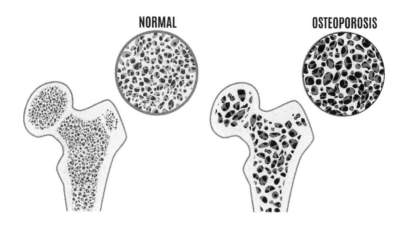

Diagram 23: Normal and porous bone.

Peak bone mass is the maximum amount of bone a person has during their life. It typically occurs in the early to mid-twenties in females and late twenties in males. Females usually have lower peak bone than males, and Caucasian people usually have lower peak bone mass than black populations.

Onset of Osteoporosis

Estradiol levels steadily decline from age forty to fifty (perimenopause), then sharply fall after menopause. The decline in estradiol at menopause directly correlates with the onset of osteoporosis. Women lose about 10 percent of their bone mass in the first five years after menopause.

The annual rate of postmenopausal bone loss is about 1.3 to 1.5 percent. Eventually, fractures occur with the slightest injury, and there is an increasing incidence of spontaneous compression fractures. By the time that people have reached their eighties and nineties, bones have become irreversibly weak and porous.

On average, the ten-year cumulative loss is 9.1 percent at the femoral neck and 10.6 percent at the lumbar spine.

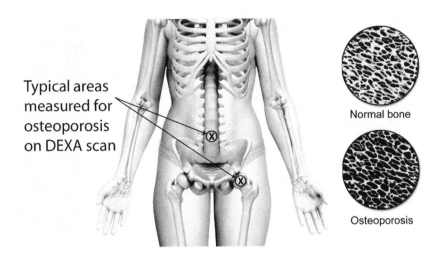

Typical areas measured for osteoporosis on DEXA scan

Normal bone

Osteoporosis

Diagram 24: Femoral neck and lumbar spine.

Estradiol concentrations correlate with and can predict the risk of fractures. Estradiol levels of less than 5 pg/ml have been associated with a 2.5-fold increase in hip and vertebral fractures in older women.

Men naturally convert a portion of their testosterone to estradiol, which is necessary to maintain bone structure. Bone loss increases in men after andropause due to lower levels of testosterone.

Estradiol: A Key Regulator of Bone Remodeling in Adults

Over eighty years ago, Fuller Albright, a renowned American endocrinologist, recognized that osteoporosis is associated with estrogen deficiency.[62] After decades of data and research, we know that estradiol is the key hormonal regulator of bone metabolism in women and men.[63]

Bone tissue is alive. Throughout our lives, our bones are constantly being remodeled. Bone tissue gets broken down (resorbed) and reconstructed by interacting with many critically important hormones and molecules. About 10 percent of the skeleton is replaced every year. Normal human adults remodel a particular area of bone in about six to nine months.[64]

Estradiol plays a crucial role in the remodeling of bone by its action on critically important cells and molecules that are involved in the bone remodeling process. When estradiol is low, the bone resorption (breakdown) rate is greater than the reconstruction rate, with a net result of osteoporosis.

A significantly higher risk of hip fracture results from a shortened lifetime exposure to estradiol, such as late menarche (onset of the menstrual cycle) or early menopause. Earlier menarche has been associated with a slightly better protective effect than later menopause. Late puberty (which results from low circulating estradiol levels) has been associated with a non-maximum bone mass and higher fracture risk.[65, 66, 67, 68]

Effects of Osteoporosis

Osteoporosis has no obvious symptoms until bones break, unlike weak muscles, tendons, and ligaments. The physical profile of men and women through the decades clearly shows the effects of the degenerative changes which occur with aging. By the eighth and ninth decade, a person with a once upright, poised posture has steadily become hunched, stooped, and frail.

As we age, our bones weaken to such a degree that fractures can occur with minor stress or even spontaneously. After the fracture heals, there is usually chronic pain and decreased ability to carry out everyday activities.

The cumulative effects of osteoporosis and compression fractures can devastate a person's independence, quality of life, and finances. People with fractures and frailty resulting from osteoporosis often develop depression due to a lack of freedom.

Spine

The spine supports the upper body. Weakening of the bones of the vertebra results in severe pain and disability. As a result of the aging spine:

- The posture becomes stooped and hunched.
- There is an increased risk of spinal stenosis and sciatica, resulting in pain and numbness due to nerve impingement.
- The lower vertebrae (L1–L5) bear most of the upper body's weight; compression of the lumbar spine can cause fractures, due to the weakened bones being compressed from the body's weight. This is one of the most debilitating effects of osteoporosis and poor bone remodeling.
- Cervical spine fractures result in tremendous pain, weakness, disability of the upper body, and risk of spinal cord damage.
- Compression of the vertebrae (bones of the spines) leads to a change in the spine's alignment, resulting in loss of height.
- Fractures in the thoracic spine affect air movement in the lungs—every thoracic vertebral body collapse results in nearly 10 percent loss of lung volume.

Aging Spine

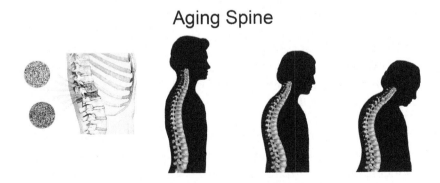

Diagram 25: Aging spine.

Falls and Fractures

The risk of falls increases with age due to a combination of degenerative changes in the body. The cardiovascular system, nervous system, muscles, ligaments, and joints undergo age-related deterioration, increasing the risk of falls. In youth, relatively heavy-impact falls have little or no (perceptible) consequences; a slight trip or fall in an older adult results in fractures that can dramatically affect the quality of life.

The most common fractures due to falls are pelvic, hip, femur, wrist, forearms, and shoulders.

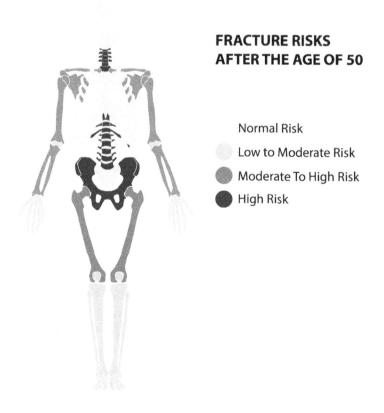

FRACTURE RISKS AFTER THE AGE OF 50

Normal Risk

Low to Moderate Risk

Moderate To High Risk

High Risk

Diagram 26

Pelvic and Hip Fractures

Hip and pelvic fractures are common in the elderly, and create a medical dilemma. These fractures are associated with a poor quality of life and high mortality. However, surgery in elderly people with multiple other age-related chronic diseases often carries a higher risk of mortality than the fracture itself. In such cases where surgery is not a safe option, patients suffer great pain and debility for the rest of their lives. Due to the debility from the fractures, it is often unsafe for patients to return home, and so, nursing home placement is required.

Hip and pelvic fractures are also associated with deep vein thrombosis and pulmonary embolism (blood clots), leading to increased mortality.

Facial Bones and Teeth

As we age, the shape of our faces changes. There is a tendency for the jaw to grow forward, losing the youthful definition. Although teeth are technically not bone, they are supported by the bones in the jaw—the jawbone supports and anchors teeth. When the jawbone becomes less dense, tooth shifting or loss can occur.

Ears

Three tiny bones in the middle ear play an essential role in amplifying sound. Osteoporosis impacts these small ear bones (auditory ossicles), causing weakness and deterioration. Osteoporosis can increase the risk of developing hearing loss. An investigation in Taiwan compared 10,660 people with osteoporosis to 31,980 without osteoporosis. Results showed that people with osteoporosis were 76 percent more likely to develop sudden hearing loss. Women with osteoporosis were 87 percent more likely to develop sudden hearing loss than men.[69]

How Estradiol Regulates Bone Remodeling

Ounce for an ounce, healthy bone is stronger than steel. The complex and elaborate structure of bone is composed of a mineral matrix for strength and collagen fibers for flexibility and resilience. The fracture risk is inversely proportional to the estrogen level in postmenopausal women.

Osteoblasts, osteocytes, and *osteoclasts* are the primary specialized cells in bone development and remodeling. All three of these bone cells have estradiol receptors, and estradiol regulates bone metabolism by interacting with these cells. Many other essential immune system proteins (cytokines) and growth factors are vital in regulating bone remodeling. Estradiol directly influences them.

Here is a closer look at each of these cells.

Osteoblasts are cells that secrete new bone and build the bone matrix.

- Low estradiol decreases the number of osteoblasts.
- Estrogen promotes the activity of osteoblasts.
- When estrogen levels drop after menopause, the osteoblasts cannot effectively produce bone.
- Estrogen also affects osteoblast activity in men, preventing bone loss.
- Therefore, estrogen deficiency leads to inadequate bone formation.

Osteoclasts are cells that resorb bone so that the body can make new bone.

- Low estradiol increases the number of osteoclasts.
- Estradiol directly acts upon osteoclasts (through estradiol receptors) and decreases their bone breakdown effects.[70, 71, 72]
- Estradiol indirectly affects osteoclasts by suppressing other protein molecules that are involved with bone breakdown.

- Estradiol promotes apoptosis (programmed cell death) of osteoclasts. The lack of estradiol results in a longer life-span of osteoclasts, leading to increased bone loss.[73]

Osteocytes are cells that trigger bone remodeling by sensing mechanical strain.

- Estrogen replacement with weight-bearing and resistance exercises after menopause have been shown to build bone strength.[74, 75]

- Weight-bearing and mechanical strain increase osteocyte activity, which increases bone maintenance and regulation. The weightlessness in space travel is associated with reduced bone mineral density and accelerated bone loss.[76]

Cytokines are small proteins associated with the immune system that also play a critical role in bone remodeling, especially during bone injury.[77]

- Estradiol suppresses the secretion of cytokines that are involved in bone resorption and alters the balance of the different cytokines, favoring bone building.[78]

- Estradiol is involved in controlling the number of specific immune cells. Loss of estradiol causes the expansion of T-cells (immune cells), leading to rapid bone loss.

Diagnosing Osteoporosis

Osteopenia occurs before osteoporosis. A DEXA (dual-energy x-ray absorptiometry) scan evaluates bone density. Osteopenia means the bone density is between 1 and 2.5 standard deviations below that of a young adult. This is also reported as a T-score between -1 and -2.5.

Osteoporosis is defined as the bone density of 2.5 standard deviations below that of a young adult or a T-score less than -2.5.

Severe osteoporosis means a T-score is less than -2.5 and a fragility fracture.

Osteoporosis Effects on Society

By 2025, more than 3 million cases of osteoporotic fractures will occur annually, bringing with them an estimated cost of 25.3 billion dollars. Medicare pays the bulk of the treatment cost of these fractures. There is an additional non-fracture osteoporosis cost of several billion dollars for drug treatments. Furthermore, patients and the healthcare system spend additional billions of dollars treating the side effects of the inadequate, harsh medications offered to treat osteoporosis.

The United States is not the only country treating osteoporosis poorly. In the United Kingdom, about 3 million people have osteoporosis. Above 500,000 people with fragility fractures go to the hospital in the United Kingdom each year, representing an estimated cost to the National Health Service of £4.4 billion a year.

Other factors contributing to osteoporosis include alcoholism, anorexia, hypothyroidism, kidney disease, non-steroidal anti-inflammatories, glucocorticosteroids, chemotherapy, SSRIs (antidepressants), and seizure medications.

When osteoporosis's effects accumulate to debility and fractures, the damage is difficult to repair.

Bisphosphonates—Non-Hormonal Medical Therapy for Osteoporosis

Bisphosphonates are a class of drugs commonly used to treat osteoporosis. They are said to reduce the breakdown/resorption of bone by encouraging osteoclasts (cells that break down bone) to undergo cell death, thereby slowing bone loss. However, bisphosphonates create their own problems.

Bone tissue undergoes constant remodeling and is kept in balance by osteoblasts that are creating bone and osteoclasts that are destroying bone. Long-term use of bisphosphonates results in over-suppression of bone turnover, which can make bone brittle over time and has been linked to unusual fractures: "bisphosphonate fractures."

The most remarkable side effects are osteonecrosis (bone cell death that is due to loss of blood supply) of the jaw, joint and muscle pain, and esophagitis.

Intravenous bisphosphonates can result in fevers and a flu-like syndrome due to the activation of immune cells. Prolonged use of bisphosphonates suppresses the immune system.

Bisphosphonates have an affinity for calcium and accumulate in the bone. They remain in the body for decades, as it cannot metabolize them. They are either eventually excreted by the kidneys or are deposited within the bones. The amount of drug within the bone will accumulate with use, and there is no known method of removing it.

Hormone Therapy for Osteoporosis

Through its effects on multiple cells and molecules, estradiol allows the complex structure and crystal lattice of the bone to be maintained. Numerous studies compared bone mineral density in women on hormone replacement therapy versus those who were not. These studies reiterated that long-term prevention of bone loss by the presence of ample estrogen has vital medical, social, and economic implications.[79]

A balanced diet with vitamin D, vitamin K2, and calcium without adequate estradiol has minimum benefits.

Women

Estradiol replacement is the safest and most natural solution for preventing osteoporosis. Osteoporosis starts (at least) around ten years before menopause, when estradiol levels begin to decline significantly. Therefore, it is important to maintain healthy normal levels to optimize bone preservation when replacing estradiol.

Men

Men with normal testosterone levels produce an adequate amount of estradiol for bone remodeling and preservation. Healthcare providers treating men for osteoporosis strive to keep the blood levels of testosterone in normal, healthy ranges so that the body can maintain a healthy level of estradiol through normal internal conversion.

Osteoarthritis and Joint Pain

Osteoarthritis

Osteoarthritis is an age-related degenerative joint disease. It causes pain and stiffness in the affected joints. Commonly affected joints bear the most weight, such as the knees, hips, and lower back.

Joints that involve the most movement, such as the joints in the hands and feet, eventually have typical osteoarthritic changes (usually accelerating after about age fifty), affecting daily activities and chores and reducing the quality of life.

Osteoarthritis starts with cartilage deterioration. As the cartilage—a tough, flexible tissue between the ends of two bones—degenerates, the ends of the bones rub against each other, causing stiffness. The body attempts to repair the damage by creating bone to replace the deteriorated cartilage. In some cases, bone spurs (protruding pieces of bone) are formed, which cause further stiffening, pain, and swelling, due to inflammation of the surrounding structures (tendons, ligaments, synovium, etc.).[80, 81]

OSTEOARTHRITIS

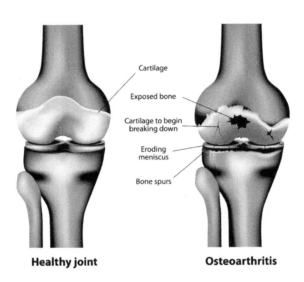

Diagram 27: Osteoarthritis in the knee joint.

Estrogen maintains healthy joints by:

- Maintaining the structure of the cartilage in the joints (articular cartilage).
- Maintaining proper bone remodeling, including the ends of the bone (subchondral bone), which are connected to cartilage.
- Reducing inflammation in the joint space.
- Promoting the production of healthy joint fluid (synovial fluid).

8

SKELETAL MUSCLE, TENDONS, AND LIGAMENTS

We become predictably weaker and senile every decade after menopause and andropause. In addition to other aging processes, our bones become porous and weak; our muscles, tendons, ligaments, and joints degenerate. A large part of this weakness is preventable with correct and timely intervention.

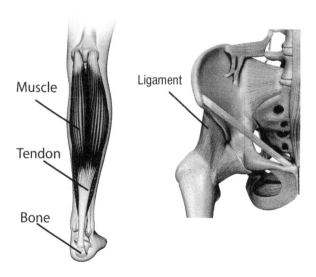

Diagram 28: Bone, muscle, tendon, and ligament.

Skeletal muscles, ligaments, and tendons hold our skeleton together, which provides stability, movement, and mobility. The combination of muscle weakness, stiff tendons and ligaments, and degenerative joints results in loss of strength and the emergence of frailty with aging.

For almost 100 years, we have known that estradiol prevents osteoporosis. In recent years, studies consistently showed that estradiol, directly and indirectly, regulates the function of muscles, tendons, ligaments, joint tissue, and cartilage. These structures' cells have estradiol receptors.

Estradiol improves muscle mass and strength. It increases the collagen content of tendons and ligaments, maintaining strength while decreasing their stiffness. Also, estradiol contributes to normal joint cartilage formation and joint fluid (synovial fluid) production.

In addition to directly acting on the cells of muscles, tendons, and ligaments, estradiol is essential in regulating countless chemical processes. These processes are required to maintain the normal metabolic function within musculoskeletal system structures.

Bones weaken as we age, but we can neither feel the strength level of our bones, nor sense pain from osteoporosis until we suffer from a fracture or related consequences of weakened bones. Other degenerative processes, including sarcopenia (muscle weakness), osteoarthritis (degeneration of joints), and tendon and ligament weakness cause symptoms that impact the quality of life.

Not everyone ages the same way. Genetic and lifestyle factors, such as diet and exercise, play a role in the manner and speed of aging, but the further that we age beyond menopause and andropause, the less that we benefit from diet and exercise alone.

Menopause and andropause are associated with an increased risk of musculoskeletal injury and accelerated bone and muscle wasting.[82]

As the body ages:

- Muscles become weaker, resulting in low energy and easy fatigability.

- Tendons and ligaments become stiffer and more brittle, reducing flexibility.

- Synovial (joint) fluid reduces, impacting joints' smooth mobility.

- Movement becomes progressively slower due to stiff ligaments, tendons, joints, and muscle weakness.

- Muscles, tendons, and ligaments respond in a complex way to brain signals to maintain balance and equilibrium. In addition to the slower nervous system response from aging, muscles become weak; tendons and ligaments become stiff; and maintaining balance becomes more difficult.

- Risk of falls increases.

- Reduced movement accumulates in increased weight gain.

Direct Effect of Estradiol on Skeletal Muscle

Skeletal muscle is the muscle attached to bones for movement and strength. The steady increase in skeletal muscle degeneration starts in perimenopause and further increases after menopause. Sarcopenia is the loss of muscle as a natural part of aging, and it results in physical debility, loss of quality of life, and financial costs.

Estradiol is essential for comprehensively maintaining muscle mass and strength. However, having low estradiol levels reduces muscle strength and regeneration. Studies show that prolonged estrogen insufficiency results in muscle atrophy in a time-dependent manner.

Satellite cells are cells that support muscle cells. Their expansion, differentiation, and self-renewal depend on normal levels of estradiol. As a result, low estradiol levels ultimately compromise muscle regeneration.[83]

In muscle tissue, estradiol acts directly at the DNA level to promote the production of muscle proteins, thus preserving muscle mass. Studies demonstrate that postmenopausal women using estrogen replacement therapy have a more significant muscle-building response to exercise.

Estrogen influences the ability of muscles to contract and plays a significant role in stimulating muscle repair and regenerative processes, including those related to post-exercise muscle injury.[84]

Estradiol exerts its protective effects in numerous ways, including acting as an antioxidant, thus limiting oxidative damage. In addition, it stabilizes the cell membrane and regulates other genes and molecules that are required for repair and the regenerative process.

Testosterone and Muscles

As established previously, men naturally convert a portion of their testosterone to estradiol. However, testosterone also has additional benefits in muscle protein synthesis, which is why males tend to have a larger and stronger muscle mass than females. The female metabolic system does *not* handle high testosterone levels as a male does. High testosterone levels in women increase *metabolic syndrome*, which consists of insulin resistance, high cholesterol, and high blood pressure.

In women, progesterone *enhances* the estradiol effect of muscle protein synthesis.[85] Women with healthy adrenal glands and correct replacement of estradiol and progesterone continue to make enough testosterone throughout life.

Oral Contraceptives and the Musculoskeletal System

Oral contraceptives stop the ovarian production of estradiol, leaving the body with very low estradiol levels. This low-circulating level of estradiol inhibits protein synthesis in tendons, ligaments, and muscle tissue.

Studies on Estradiol and Skeletal Muscle

There is no substitute for the lack of estradiol. Numerous studies have shown that, no matter how much women may participate in resistance training and eat well, without sufficient estradiol, the degenerative process will continue, and muscle loss accelerates.

There are exhaustive medical studies on the direct effects of estradiol on skeletal muscle, including its impact on muscle mass and function; below are a few examples:

- An Australian study compared 840 postmenopausal women: 581 not on estradiol replacement and 259 on estradiol. Muscle cross-sectional analysis found that muscle cross-sectional area (CSA) and grip strength were *greater* in estradiol users than in non-users.[86]

- Researchers at UCLA studied animals after the surgical removal of ovaries. Twenty-four weeks of estrogen deficiency resulted in a 10 percent *decrease* in muscle strength and an 18 percent *decrease* in muscle fiber cross-sectional area. Replacing estradiol caused a return of *muscle strength*.[87] The studies also demonstrated that the *response to exercise and muscle recovery* was much greater in animals that were receiving estradiol.

- A study measuring muscle fiber protein synthesis in women taking estradiol replacement therapy showed that women who were taking estradiol had a better response to resistance exercise than those who were not.[88, 89]

- A Finnish study published in 2009 studied sixteen postmenopausal identical twins, comparing thigh muscle composition, lower body muscle power (by measuring vertical jump height), knee extension strength, hand grip, maximal walking speed, and habitual walking.

  One of each twin took estrogen replacement therapy, and the other did not. Maximal walking speed, vertical jump height, thigh muscle cross-sectional area (CSA), and relative muscle area were greater in the estrogen replacement therapy twins than in their sisters. There was no measurable difference in habitual walking. Serum estradiol levels were more than five times higher in the estrogen replacement therapy user.[90]

- In 2001, Finnish researchers split eighty postmenopausal women into four groups:

    1. Exercise only,

    2. Hormone replacement therapy only,

    3. Exercise plus hormone replacement therapy, or

    4. No hormone therapy or exercise for one year.

    Exercise alone was less effective than hormone replacement therapy in maintaining muscle mass. As expected, hormone replacement therapy and exercise improved muscle mass and function more than either hormone replacement therapy or exercise alone.[91]

- A study compared young women using oral contraceptives versus those not using them. The day after performing specific leg exercises, muscle fiber breakdown and synthesis were measured. Muscle fiber protein synthesis was lower in women on oral contraceptives. The positive effects of testosterone were also reduced in women on oral contraceptives. In conclusion, oral contraceptive use had an inhibiting effect on muscle protein synthesis.[92]

Indirect Effects of Estradiol on Skeletal Muscle

Consider the many critical metabolic effects of estradiol on skeletal muscles:

1. Loss of estradiol results in the harmful increase of hydrogen peroxide (H_2O_2) production within the tiny, energy-producing organelles (mitochondria) in cells.[93]

2. Low estradiol results in decreased production of antioxidant proteins (glutathione peroxidase, catalase, and superoxide dismutase) within the muscle cells.[94]

3. Low estradiol results in impaired insulin sensitivity.[95]

Because of the metabolic derangements from low estradiol, muscles fatigue more quickly and regenerate less, causing an ongoing cycle of weakness and debility. Replacement with normal estradiol levels restores the muscle cells' normal metabolic function.[96, 97]

Estradiol's Effects on Tendons and Ligaments

First, a few definitions:

Tendons attach muscle to bone and consist of tough, fibrous connective tissue that is made of collagen (~65–80 percent) and elastin (~1–2 percent).

Ligaments attach bone to bone; for example, bones in the spine, shoulders, knees, feet, ankles, hands, wrists, elbows, etc. Ligaments are made of collagen (~80 percent) and elastin (~5 percent).

Tendons & Ligaments

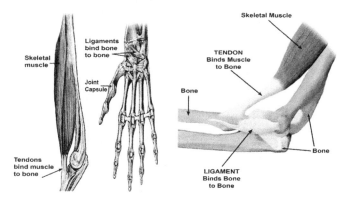

Diagram 29

Tendons and ligaments are incredibly tough and resilient structures, which are constructed with the correct balance of flexibility, laxity, and strength.

The extremely high levels of estradiol in pregnancy allow the changes needed for the woman to carry and deliver a baby. The tendons and ligaments in women have a different collagen to elastin ratio than men. It makes sense that women have laxer joints, which facilitates healthy childbirth and recovery. However, as more women participate in traditionally male sports, the physiological effects of estrogen contribute to decreases in power and performance and make women more prone to catastrophic ligament injury.

Many studies compare premenopausal women on oral contraceptives (a low estradiol state) to premenopausal women with a natural ovarian cycle that produces significantly more estradiol. Normal estradiol levels result in a *higher* level of collagen synthesis after exercise, which is beneficial for joint integrity and maintenance.[98]

Estradiol replacement therapy in postmenopausal women increases tendon collagen and elastin synthesis, which helps to maintain structural balance and reduce stiffness.[99]

Studies Demonstrating Estradiol Effects on Ligaments and Tendons

The profound impact of estradiol's effect on collagen synthesis prompted numerous well-designed studies in academic centers worldwide to conduct further investigation. For example:

- Multiple studies demonstrated that premenopausal women on oral contraceptives (low estradiol state) had decreased exercise-stimulated collagen synthesis. After one hour of kicking exercise, women on oral contraceptives had no change in collagen synthesis, while women with normal hormone levels had doubled their patellar (knee) tendon collagen production.[100, 101, 102]

- A well-designed study from Denmark showed that pre-menopausal women with a consistently low estrogen level due to oral contraceptives had decreased collagen synthesis. However, in postmenopausal women, estrogen replacement therapy, which provided a moderate daily rise in estrogen, was linked with *increased* tendon collagen synthesis. The study also showed that, in postmenopausal women on estradiol replacement therapy, collagen incorporation into the patellar tendon was 47 percent higher compared with the control group (who were not on estradiol replacement therapy).[103]

- Estradiol's pivotal role in maintaining homeostasis (structural equilibrium) of female connective tissue was demonstrated through sophisticated studies using isotopes, MRI imaging, electron microscopy, and ultrasound recording. Menopausal women who were using estradiol showed significantly improved tendon synthesis, structure, and biomechanical properties than postmenopausal women who were not using estradiol.

- Estradiol was shown to increase the effects of insulin-like growth factor (IGF-1), a hormone involved in countless functions, including the structural maintenance of the musculoskeletal system. IGF-1 *increases* tendon collagen synthesis and incorporation into the tendons, maintaining tendon structure and strength.[104, 105]

Summary

- Our muscles, tendons, ligaments, and joints degenerate as we age. Mobility and quality of life continuously decline. A large part of this is preventable with correct and timely hormone replacement therapy.

- Postmenopausal women and men after andropause have a higher rate of muscle protein breakdown than synthesis, resulting in a rapid decrease in muscle mass and strength, leading to age-related frailty.

- Muscle cells have estradiol receptors. Estradiol improves muscle protein production, increasing muscle mass and strength.[106]

- Estradiol increases the collagen and elastin content of tendons and ligaments, improving strength and reducing stiffness.

- Estradiol contributes to normal joint cartilage formation and joint fluid (synovial fluid) production.

- Postmenopausal women using estrogen replacement therapy have a greater muscle-building response to exercise.[107]

- Estradiol acts as an antioxidant, thus limiting oxidative damage, stabilizing the cell membrane, and regulating other genes and molecules required for the repair and regenerative process.

- Estradiol has anti-degradative properties at the level of cartilage and increases synovial fluid production, which helps to maintain healthy joints.

- There is no substitute for lack of estradiol. Men convert a significant portion of testosterone to estradiol to achieve the benefits of estradiol on the musculoskeletal system.

9

ESTRADIOL AND CARDIOVASCULAR HEALTH

Under the strong influence of Big Pharma, the way that mainstream medicine handles cardiovascular disease prevention is among the most unfortunate disservices done to women and men. The cardioprotective effects of estradiol are well recognized and accepted in the world of science and medicine.

Before menopause, women have a relatively low risk of developing cardiovascular disease. After menopause, the risk dramatically increases, making cardiovascular disease the *number one* cause of death among women and the greatest source of revenue for the pharmaceutical and medical industry.

Facts Known for Decades:

- For over seventy years, we have recognized premenopausal women have a lower incidence of cardiovascular disease than men. Prior to menopause, women have less heart disease than men; after menopause, the risk is similar.

- For over fifty years, we have recognized that estradiol lowers LDL.

- In women, the risk of insulin resistance, lipid disorders, and hypertension all increase after menopause.

Thousands of laboratory studies throughout the world, over many decades, consistently defined estradiol's cardioprotective effects on cellular and molecular mechanisms of the cardiovascular system.

Estradiol and the Introduction of Synthetic Hormones

In the 1930s, scientists discovered how to produce estradiol. Soon afterward, Big Pharma took over and developed an alternative and patentable version of estradiol.

Big Pharma convinced physicians—and those in power, including the FDA—that synthetic (molecularly altered and fake) estrogen is the same or even better than the bioidentical estrogen (estradiol) that a woman's body makes. Big Pharma and physicians ignored that oral estrogen and oral progesterone have side effects.

The synthetic, non-human version of estrogen introduced by a major pharmaceutical company was conjugated equine estrogen (CEE), also known as Premarin® (discussed in more detail in earlier chapters). In 1941, CEE (Premarin®) became available for prescriptions.

As mentioned in chapter 1, in the 1970s, synthetic progesterone medroxyprogesterone acetate (also known as MPA or Provera®) was introduced by the same company that made Premarin®, and its purpose was to balance the effects of the estrogens in CEE (Premarin®).

Again, Prempro® comes from combining Premarin® with MPA, which is fake progesterone.

- Premarin® (CEE) is synthetic estrogen.
- Provera® (MPA) is synthetic progesterone.
- Prempro® is a combination of **Prem**arin and **Pro**vera.

Harmful Studies with Misleading Results

The government required studies before Premarin® and Prempro® (synthetic estradiol and progesterone) could be accepted as "standard of care" for the prevention of cardiovascular disease. This led to the *Heart and Estrogen/Progestin Replacement Study (HERS)* and the *Women's Health Initiative (WHI)* study.

Both studies showed an *increase* rather than a *decrease* in cardiovascular disease in women who were taking Premarin and Prempro. The results from these studies were shocking and contradicted decades of laboratory research consistently showing that estradiol was cardioprotective. Further analysis of the HERS and WHI study uncovered many severe and significant flaws in both studies:

- None of the major studies that showed that estrogen was linked to cardiovascular disease used *human* estrogen in normal human ranges. The WHI study and HERS used Premarin®, which is extracted from the urine of pregnant horses and does not contain significant levels of estradiol (the primary human estrogen).

- The studies used Premarin® by mouth. Any estrogen by mouth causes an increased risk for blood clots. (See the next section, "First Pass Metabolism," for more information.)

- Provera® was used in both studies and has many adverse effects on the body. Its effects on the human body are in stark contrast to those of the natural hormone that it was supposed to replace. Natural (bioidentical) progesterone in normal (physiological) ranges has universal protective effects on the body.

First Pass Metabolism

First pass metabolism is a vital concept. Anything you put in your mouth must go through the liver to be broken down before it enters the blood circulation. Blood from the circulation also passes through the liver for constant ongoing surveillance, but through a different route. When the liver is exposed to estrogen from the mouth, it does not account for the fact that this "high concentration" is not the true blood concentration. The liver makes clotting proteins corresponding to the concentration of estrogen it detects. Therefore, oral estrogen causes the liver to produce abnormally high clotting proteins, increasing the risk of blood clots.

Estrogen applied to the skin goes directly into the blood through the skin. After being dispersed in the blood, it then enters the hepatic (liver) circulation. This is the actual blood concentration of the drug and the concentration to which the liver and every other organ supplied by the blood will be exposed to.

The fact that estrogen by mouth causes blood clots has been well known since the 1960s, and prompted the *Nurses' Health Study*, which was an uncontrolled study and did not have much credibility as the results were conflicting, and the study design was weak.

As mentioned in the previous section, Premarin® does not contain any significant amount of estradiol; it contains many other (quite different) types of estrogens than those found in premenopausal women. Also, Premarin has a large amount of estrone, the predominant type of estrogen in postmenopausal women that is associated with clot formation.

Even when estradiol is taken by mouth, it converts to estrone in the liver and promotes the clotting mechanism.[108] This risk does not happen when estradiol is used and applied topically.[109]

As a result of a chain of colossal bad medical decisions, women and men have, and continue to suffer, from age-related cardiovascular disease, a state that can be significantly curtailed with correct hormone replacement therapy.

Estrogen Benefits on the Cardiovascular System

The cardiovascular system consists of the heart and the blood vessels that circulate blood throughout the body. The degeneration of the cardiovascular system results in:

- Decreased contraction strength and relaxation of the heart muscles (leading to congestive heart failure).

- Stiffening and narrowing of blood vessels (contributing to high blood pressure, heart attacks, and stroke).

- Increased free radicals and inflammatory proteins (causing deterioration of blood vessel walls and muscle injury).

Inflammation and Oxidative Stress

We know that aging is associated with oxidative stress from free radicals[110] and inflammation. Estradiol has anti-inflammatory and antioxidant effects, demonstrated in numerous studies.[111]

Estradiol acts as an antioxidant by upregulating the DNA production of a critically important enzyme called endothelial nitric oxide synthase, which increases blood flow by dilating blood vessels and decreasing superoxide production.[112]

Reperfusion Injury

During a heart attack, cardiac muscle is injured due to the lack of blood flow and oxygen. This suffocation of heart muscle triggers immediate compensation mechanisms. Once blood flow is reestablished, there is tissue damage from the increased local production of inflammatory proteins and free radicals. Estrogen protects against reperfusion injury through its anti-inflammatory and antioxidant effects.[113]

Smooth Muscle

There are three types of muscles in the body: *Smooth muscle, cardiac muscle, and skeletal muscle.* Skeletal muscle is the muscle attached to bone and allows movement. (See chapter 8 on skeletal muscle for more information.)

Other than skeletal muscle, smooth muscle makes up most of our insides and what are described as hollow structures, such as blood vessels, intestines, digestive tract, uterus, bladder, lungs, reproductive organs, as well as around the eyes and various other places. Smooth muscle is not involved in voluntary physical movement but has critical, life-sustaining functions.

The health and integrity of blood vessels is paramount to our health and wellness. Blood vessels carrying blood throughout the body have a tubular structure made of several layers with distinct properties. Vascular smooth muscle cells are a crucial component of blood vessels. Estradiol plays an important role in maintaining the balanced production and function of all types of smooth muscle cells.

The degeneration of smooth muscle structures in the body results in the slow deterioration of our health and wellness. Women have vaginal dryness after menopause, which is directly correlated with low estradiol. Vaginal dryness is a critical indicator that smooth muscle structures in other parts of the body are degenerating.

Vascular Function and Nitric Oxide

Aging increases vascular constriction, decreases relaxation, and decreases flow-mediated vasodilation (appropriate dilation of the blood vessel with blood flow). As a result, blood pressure increases, and vessels become damaged over time. Estradiol replacement increases vascular flow and reduces blood flow resistance.[114]

Nitroglycerine is the medication given to patients with known coronary artery disease undergoing an angina episode. Constriction of blood vessels in the heart leads to "suffocation" of the surrounding heart muscle, causing significant pain (angina). Nitroglycerine taken under the tongue immediately gets into the bloodstream and converts to nitrous oxide, relaxing the constricted blood vessel and relieving the pain. Estrogen is known to naturally enhance nitrous oxide production, which relaxes blood vessel walls.[115]

Studies on women have shown that estradiol therapy after menopause improves relaxation of blood vessel walls.[116, 117] While estradiol increases nitrous oxide production, causing relaxation of blood vessels, the conjugated equine estrogens (CEE) in Premarin® *impair* nitrous oxide production.[118, 119, 120, 121]

Hyperglycemia, Metabolic Syndrome, and Cardiovascular Disease

High blood glucose negatively affects blood vessels, changing their structure and causing increased thickness, which leads to stiffer, less healthy blood vessels.[122] Studies have shown that estradiol prevents hyperglycemia-induced proliferation (overgrowth) of vascular smooth muscle cells.[123] Estrones (which, again, are the main estrogens in CEE [Premarin®]), do not offer this positive, protective effect.[124]

Studies have consistently shown that estrogen plays a pivotal role in controlling energy balance and glucose homeostasis via a diverse set of mechanisms.[125] Clinical trials and animal studies proved that the drop in estrogen at menopause sets off rapid changes in whole-body metabolism, fat distribution, and insulin function.

Women with metabolic syndrome (abdominal obesity, insulin resistance, and dyslipidemia) are at especially high risk for cardiovascular disease (CVD). The prevalence of the metabolic syndrome increases after menopause and explains the increased abdominal fat, increased cholesterol, and insulin resistance which starts to occur as menopause approaches. This change is directly related to the fall in estradiol.[126]

Atherosclerosis and Dyslipidemia

Atherosclerosis is an age-related disease of arteries where plaque builds up on the inner lining of the blood vessel walls, causing arterial narrowing. If part of a plaque breaks off, it can travel to smaller arteries and block blood flow, causing tissue damage, including devastating outcomes such as a heart attack or stroke.

Menopause is associated with the acceleration of atherosclerosis and deterioration of blood vessel (vascular) structure.[127] Estradiol also enhances *angiogenesis*, which is the creation of new blood vessels, thus helping to preserve tissue integrity.

LDL Cholesterol

LDL cholesterol is a vital molecule once it is in the right place. Among other essential uses, LDL cholesterol is the precursor (starting molecule) to all steroid hormones and a necessary part of cell walls, the brain, and the nervous system. When a cell anywhere in the body registers low LDL cholesterol inside it, it produces proteins to signal the liver to make more LDL cholesterol. With aging, fewer LDL cholesterol cell receptors are made by the liver, causing the LDL cholesterol levels in the blood to increase. Cholesterol-lowering medications (statins) reduce the liver response by interfering with the messenger proteins made by cells that tell the liver to produce more LDL cholesterol.

Estradiol stimulates the liver to make more cell receptors for LDL cholesterol,[128] so that it can enter the cell and become what it is supposed to rather than accumulating in the blood, combining with calcium, and depositing as plaques.

Atherosclerosis

Beyond its role in improving lipid metabolism, many studies show how estradiol plays a crucial role in curtailing the process of atherosclerosis (the building up of plaques in the arterial walls).

Atherosclerosis involves a highly complex set of events and processes involving inflammatory molecules, adhesion of white blood cells, and multiple other factors.[129] Many studies demonstrated that estradiol's physiological levels reduce the production of inflammatory proteins, block the adhesiveness of cells that contribute to plaque formation, and decrease the production of plaque-forming molecules.[130, 131, 132, 133] Multiple studies revealed how estradiol protects the lining of blood vessel walls from injury and degeneration.[134, 135, 136]

Cardiac Muscles

Enormous data and evidence confirm the cardioprotective effects of estradiol. Estradiol's impact on the heart occurs by numerous mechanisms, including genomic effects (directly acting on the cell DNA to initiate synthesis of important molecules) and non-genomic effects (acting within the cell to start numerous critical functions).

Heart muscle is the hardest working muscle in the body, as the heart never stops beating. With every heartbeat, the heart muscle contracts and relaxes. Although heart muscle contraction requires energy, heart muscle relaxation involves even more energy. Heart failure develops due to inadequate contraction or relaxation of the heart muscles.

Estradiol is a significant regulator of heart muscle cells' (cardiomyocytes') bioenergetics (metabolism and energy balance).[137, 138] Estradiol replacement has been shown to improve heart muscle (myocardial) energy production, which is critical for contraction and the relaxation of heart muscles after contraction.[139]

Numerous studies investigated estradiol's effects on preventing stress-induced cardiac cell death via multiple different key pathways within the cells.[140, 141, 142, 143, 144, 145, 146, 147, 148]

Studies confirm that estradiol protects cardiac function by stimulating the production of cardiac muscle cells (myocytes) from progenitor cells (cardiac-specific stem cells). This function is crucial for preserving cardiac function after myocardial infarction.[149, 150, 151]

Summary

- After menopause, the risk of cardiovascular disease dramatically increases.

- From clinical observations and thousands of laboratory studies, it is known that estradiol has significant cardiovascular protective effects.

- Estradiol in physiological ranges improves the function of the heart muscle so that it can contract and relax properly, preventing heart failure.

- Estradiol helps maintain proper blood vessels and smooth muscle structure.

- Estradiol improves lipid profile, increases LDL receptors, and reduces atherosclerosis.

- Estradiol helps repair cell and tissue injury by multiple mechanisms.

- The two major studies that "showed" estrogen to cause harm or no benefit used *synthetic* estrogen and *synthetic* progesterone, which have very different effects on the body than bioidentical estrogen and progesterone. The estrogen used in the studies was given by mouth, which is a risk for blood clots. Blood levels of estradiol were negligible.

- No study has used estradiol and progesterone topically in normal human ranges. It is impossible to reproduce normal human benefits using fake hormones or hormones at subnormal doses.

- Most doctors are unaware of the truth regarding estrogen because it is not taught or prioritized in their training.

- Men convert a substantial portion of testosterone to estradiol for cardioprotective effects.

10

ESTRADIOL AND PROGESTERONE EFFECTS ON THE IMMUNE SYSTEM

A healthy immune system is critical to our survival. The function of the immune system is to protect us from disease, harmful foreign substances (pathogens), cancer cells, and debris from within the body.

The immune system is one of the most complex areas in the body. Understanding a few basic components of the immune system and their roles will help you appreciate how estradiol and progesterone provide beneficial effects on the immune system.

Basic Components of the Immune System

- **Pathogens:** A pathogen is any substance that can cause disease.

- **Antigen:** An antigen (Ag) is the part of a pathogen that elicits a response from the immune system.

- **Antibodies:** These are proteins produced by specialized white blood cells in response to an antigen to fight the antigen and eliminate it from the body.

- **White blood cells (WBCs):** These are produced in the bone marrow. Also known as leukocytes and consist of several types of specialized cells involved in the immune response and fighting infection.

A few examples of white blood cells:

1. **B cells:** *A type of white blood cell that makes antibodies.*

2. **Helper T cells:** *Specialized white blood cells that help B cells produce antibodies and other white blood cells for the purpose of clearing infection.*

3. **NK cells (natural killer cells):** *Involved in clearing tumor cells and microbes.*

4. **Neutrophils and macrophages:** *Play a critical role in secreting substances to kill microbes and to engulf and eliminate diseased or damaged cells.*

5. **Dendritic cells:** *Powerful immune cells that are essential in the initiation of an immune response for the purpose of eliminating viruses and other pathogens.*

Aging and the Immune System

As we age, our immune system and defense against pathogens weaken. We produce fewer cells and corresponding proteins in response to an antigen. As a result, aging is associated with increased pneumonia, influenza, and other diseases, along with a prolonged and weaker recovery. The age-related decline in the immune system also explains why vaccines are less effective in older adults.

By the 1940s, studies established that females have an enhanced capability of producing antibodies,[152, 153] which allows effective resistance to infection, making females less susceptible to viral infections than males. Women are also less susceptible to cancer than males. However, this enhanced immune system has proven to be a disadvantage for women genetically predisposed to auto-immune diseases. An autoimmune disease occurs when the body does not recognize the difference between its own cells and foreign cells. It mounts an attack against specific body cells. Multiple sclerosis and lupus are among the more than eighty autoimmune diseases.

Over the past several decades, we have accumulated an incredible amount of knowledge on how estradiol and progesterone contribute to the function of a healthy immune system. The COVID-19 pandemic further illustrated the role of estradiol and progesterone in protecting against viruses.

In addition to destroying foreign pathogens such as bacteria, viruses, and other germs, the immune system can also recognize and destroy abnormal cells from within ourselves. The immune system is not perfect; not everything harmful is recognized or cleared by the immune system.

Protection from Pathogens

The immune system comprises three levels of defense mechanisms that a pathogen needs to cross in order to develop infection inside the body, which are **Physical and Chemical Barrier**, **Innate Immunity**, and **Acquired Immunity**.

Physical and Chemical Barrier

The physical and chemical barrier is the first line of defense and has two components:

1. **Physical barrier:** Includes the skin, cornea, mucosal surface of the digestive system, respiratory tract, and lining of the urological and genital systems.

2. **Chemical barrier:** Includes sweat, saliva, earwax, mucous, etc. More potent internal antimicrobial agents include acidic secretions, such as gastric fluid, urine, and lysozymes (in tears).

Once a pathogen breaches the skin and internal linings, two types of responses can be initiated: innate immunity or the acquired immune response.

Many molecular components (e.g., complement, cytokines, acute phase reactants) are involved in innate and acquired immunity.

Innate Immunity

Innate (natural) immunity does not require prior exposure to an antigen (i.e., immunologic memory) to be fully effective and can respond immediately to an antigen. It is also the quickest response after a pathogen has entered the body. It is inbuilt and mainly inherited.

Components include:

- *Phagocytic cells (e.g., neutrophils, monocytes, macrophages).*
- *Polymorphonuclear leukocytes.*
- *Innate lymphoid cells (e.g., natural killer [NK] cells).*

Features of the innate immune system

- Provides an immediate response to foreign antigens, involving immune cells and proteins that non-specifically recognize antigens and eliminate the associated pathogen.
- Involves circulating white blood cells (such as macrophages and neutrophils), which engulf the pathogens, release lysozymes (enzymes/proteins), and break down the pathogen.
- Stimulates production and activation of additional proteins (called complement proteins), which trigger an inflammatory response by the production of more white blood cells, accumulating at the infection site. This results in an inflammatory response that includes redness, pain, and swelling, resulting from the body fighting a local infection.

Acquired Immunity

Acquired immunity is a learned/adaptive response and the most complex type of immunity. It requires prior exposure to an antigen to be fully effective and takes time to develop after the initial encounter with a new invader. After that, the response is quick. This is the part of the immune system on which vaccines are based. The system remembers past exposures and is antigen-specific.

Acquired immunity involves B cells and T cells (specialized white blood cells). A "recognized" pathogen activates the B and T cells, which initiates a chain of events involving multiple other immune cells, proteins, and other molecules to fight the pathogen and protect the body from further attack.

Immune Response

The innate and acquired immune response involves hundreds of specialized cells and molecules that work together in an incredibly complex and sophisticated way. They engage in constant surveillance and clearance of pathogens.

A successful immune defense requires activation, regulation, and resolution of the immune response. Without regulation and balance, there would be ongoing damage to the body.

Patients who had a poor outcome from COVID-19 suffered from a cytokine storm (an overwhelming reaction of the immune system attempting to protect the body). The storm is due to excessive production of inflammatory cells (IL-1B, IL-2, IL-6, IL-8, TNF-a), leading to macrophage activation. IL-6 and macrophage activation increase C-Reactive Protein (CRP), which is a marker of disease severity.

How Estradiol and Progesterone Reduce Susceptibility to Infection

Every type of immune cell has abundant estrogen receptors. Estradiol regulates the production and maturation of immune cells. It plays a pivotal role in regulating the production of proteins involved in the immune response, enhancing the function of every component of the immune system.[154] Women produce a higher T cell response than men do. This is beneficial for fighting infection; but, as mentioned above, can be a disadvantage in certain auto-immune diseases.[155]

Women have a higher immune reactivity after viral infections and generally produce higher serum antibody concentrations after vaccination, yielding better protection. Estradiol stimulates anti-body production by B cells. Studies have shown that adult women can produce more neutralizing antibodies in viral infections, such as influenza, and have higher IgG (an essential type of antibody) production.[156]

Estradiol and progesterone both increase the number of T cells (which help fight pathogens), inhibit pro-inflammatory cytokines, and stimulate the CD4+ (specialized white blood cells) production of anti-inflammatory cytokines.

Hormone replacement therapy with estradiol in menopausal women produces a higher level of circulating B cells and greater control of inflammatory cytokines.[157]

Mechanism by which estradiol enhances the immune response

- Increases the production of hyaluronic acid, which protects the mouth cells and the nasal passage (down to the digestive tract and lungs) from the inflammatory reaction of a viral attack.

- Increases production of nasal mucus, which contains essential substances (such as mucins, electrolytes, IgA,

IgG, lysozyme, lactoferrin, and oligosaccharides) that have critical antibacterial and antiviral properties, which counteract upper respiratory tract infections.[158]

- Triggers immune cells so they can reduce the viral load by destroying and eliminating the virus.

- Activates the production of antiviral response cytokines (substances released by immune cells to help fight infection).[159]

- Increases the production of specialized white blood cells (dendritic cells), which play a critical role during inflammation.[160] Subtypes of dendritic cells produce critically important disease-fighting proteins (interferons) and other associated disease-fighting molecules.

Progesterone

Most immune cells (*including epithelial cells, macrophages, dendritic cells, lymphocytes, mast cells, and eosinophils*) have progesterone receptors. Progesterone inhibits pro-inflammatory cytokines and favors anti-inflammatory cytokines production.

Progesterone promotes pulmonary tissue repair by upregulating Amphiregulin (an important epidermal growth factor),[161] thus providing a synergistic effect, and increasing the positive effects of estradiol. Progesterone administration in menopausal women improves the outcome of pulmonary disease.[162] This is because progesterone has a pivotal role in repairing pulmonary tissue damage after viral infections, such as influenza A. Progesterone receptors are heavily active on certain white blood cells (natural killer cells), which helps with the process of self-destruction after they have engulfed a pathogen.[163]

Recent research has demonstrated that progesterone has an antiviral effect against the virus that causes COVID-19 (SARS-CoV-2).[164] This antiviral effect is believed to exist in all viral attacks, due to the common underlying mechanisms.

Estradiol and COVID-19

COVID-19 has provided an extreme example of the human response to a viral illness. Patients die from COVID-19 because of the "cytokine storm," not from damage that is due to internal viral replication.[165, 166, 167, 168]

The COVID-19 pandemic provided further knowledge on estradiol's effect on the immune system. This beneficial effect is present in all viral illnesses as the mechanism of immune protection follows a similar cascade of events.

Estradiol's beneficial effects on immune cells explain why a lower incidence of COVID-19 is observed among women than in men.[169] According to Global Health 50/50, the number of men and women who tested positive for COVID-19 is almost the same. However, a large majority of patients with severe symptoms are males, strongly supporting the observation that female hormones are helpful in the COVID-19 disease process. The data showed a two-to-one ratio worldwide when analyzing how rapidly the infection progresses and the severity of symptoms when comparing males with females.[170]

Data from multiple sources, including the Chinese State Council Information Office and Global Health 50/50, show that although male and female infection rates for COVID-19 were similar, mortality rates and vulnerability to the disease were much higher for men than women. Men are at a higher risk of a worse outcome or death, with the odds up to 2.4 times higher than women.

The International Severe Acute Respiratory and Emerging Infections Consortium (ISAREIC) observed that out of 17,000 patients in the United Kingdom, the percentage of women hospitalized was 40 percent. UK women had a 20 percent lower mortality than men. COVID-19 data from Italy, Spain, Germany, Switzerland, Belgium, and Norway showed that in all age groups from age twenty years and above, fatality rates were greater in males than females.[171]

There have been three coronavirus outbreaks. Since 2000, two other coronavirus outbreaks have occurred. The SARS-CoV emerged in China in 2002. Among 1,755 hospitalized patients in Hong Kong, the fatality rates were 13 percent in women and 22 percent in men.[172]

The Middle East Respiratory Syndrome Coronavirus (MERS-CoV) emerged in Saudi Arabia in 2012. Among 425 reported cases, the disease occurrence was lower in women (38 percent), with a fatality rate of 23 percent in women versus 52 percent in men.[173]

Premenopausal women have a better immunological response and are less susceptible to viral illnesses than men.[174] Premenopausal women also have a more efficient immune response with a less intense disease course than men and postmenopausal women.[175, 176, 177] Sepsis and multiorgan failure are rare in healthy young women with no pre-existing health conditions.[178]

ACE2 and *FURIN* are two proteins found on the surfaces of major tissues and organs (lining of the respiratory system, lungs, heart, kidney, blood vessels, liver, and digestive tract) that are the entry points for the COVID-19 virus. Experimental tests have reported that estradiol can reduce *ACE2* and *FURIN* production, potentially mitigating viral entry.[179, 180, 181]

CD4+ and CD8+ are crucial white blood cells that are necessary to fight infection. Small numbers of these cells are associated with poor prognosis in any viral illness, including COVID-19 and AIDS.[182] Estrogens enhance the local immune response by activating countless immune cells, such as phagocytes, dendritic cells, natural killer cells, and CD8+ cells. Once these cells are activated, they can fight the infection by destroying the virus and thus preventing its diffusion to the lower respiratory tract or by decreasing the viral load.[183]

Pregnancy and COVID-19

Studies of pregnant women infected with COVID-19 have shown that they did not clinically evolve to a more severe condition or outcome. A study that followed nine pregnant women who were diagnosed with COVID-19 in their third trimester and developed pneumonia reported that none needed mechanical ventilation or died.[184] Another study noted that pregnant women with COVID-19 did not develop severe respiratory symptoms compared to non-pregnant women.[185]

Based on our scientific knowledge, we believe that estradiol provides this protective effect. Progesterone is also known to have a synergistic effect on estradiol as well as direct benefits of its own.

Because estradiol is involved in reducing susceptibility to COVID-19 and its severity, research is focused on utilizing it as a therapeutic target. Several experts have discussed the positive effects of estradiol against COVID-19 infection as an adjuvant therapeutic option.[186, 187]

Estradiol's Suppressive Effect on Pro-Inflammatory Proteins

Estradiol's suppressive effect on IL-6 (a pro-inflammatory solid immune protein) is protective in many diseases. For example:

- Estrogen is known to be protective against metabolic bone disease by suppressing IL-6, thereby reducing bone resorption.

- Chronic hepatitis B, and its conversion to hepatocellular carcinoma (liver cancer) is more predominant in males. IL-6 is believed to be a key component in inflammation-associated development of hepatocellular carcinoma.[188]

- In a study of postmenopausal women with chronic hepatitis C, progression to liver fibrosis was decreased in women who took menopausal estrogen therapy compared to women who did not.[189]

Summary

- Estradiol and progesterone play a critical role in a healthy immune system. They provide balance and protection at every level of the body's immune defense system. This is another key reason that males convert a portion of testosterone to estradiol. It also explains the differences in immune response in premenopausal women and men and the decline in immune health after menopause.

- Estradiol protects the physical and chemical barriers of our immune system.

- Every immune cell has estradiol receptors. Estradiol plays a pivotal role in enhancing the innate and acquired immune system.

- Survival from COVID-19 clearly showed an advantage of premenopausal women over postmenopausal women and men.

- Estradiol reduces inflammation. Every disease that is exacerbated by increased inflammatory proteins is less severe with physiological levels of estradiol.

- Progesterone inhibits **pro-inflammatory** cytokines and favors the production of **anti-inflammatory cytokines.**

- Progesterone administration in menopausal women has also been shown to improve the outcome of pulmonary disease.

11

TESTOSTERONE IN MEN

Testosterone belongs to a class of hormones called androgens and is the hormone that defines male characteristics. It is the primary sex steroid in males and contributes to numerous aspects of physical and mental health and well-being.

In males, testosterone typically peaks between ages twenty and thirty, after which time the levels start declining. Testosterone levels decrease by about 1 percent yearly from age thirty to forty. After age fifty, men gradually begin feeling the effects of low testosterone. Each decade after that, there is a noticeable ongoing decline in physical and mental health.

Some of the changes of aging that are directly due to the decline in testosterone include:

- Change in body composition, with more fat and less muscle being present.
- Osteoporosis accumulates with posture changes and loss of height.
- Loss of libido and erectile dysfunction.
- A decline in cognition, memory, mental sharpness, and spatial awareness.
- Increase in coronary artery disease and cardiovascular events.[190]

- Hypertension and dyslipidemia (imbalance of lipids such as cholesterol and triglycerides).

- Mood changes, depression, and anxiety.

- Lower confidence, enthusiasm, and motivation.

- Easy fatigability and low energy.

- Poor sleep quality.

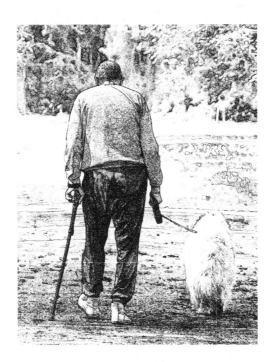

Diagram 30

The testes make most of the testosterone; the adrenal glands create the rest. As discussed before, unlike women, men do not have a sharp drop in their dominant hormone (testosterone) production that results in menopausal-like symptoms. Instead, the levels decrease over time. Men begin to age rapidly when testosterone levels are below optimum levels, just as women age after menopause.

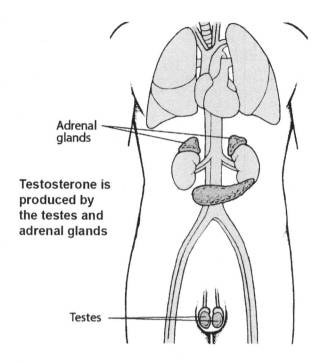

Diagram 31: Testes and adrenal glands.

After being produced in the testes and adrenal glands, testosterone circulates in the blood, bound by unique proteins called SHBG (Sex Hormone Binding Globulins), which are made in the liver. About 2 percent of the testosterone is free (unbound to SHBH) and is the more active (or bioavailable) form.

Testosterone is converted to estrogen outside the testes, which has many vital functions for men. An enzyme called 5-alpha reductase converts about 10 percent of testosterone to DHT (dihydrotestosterone), a more potent androgen form. It is the androgen responsible for male pattern baldness in men and women.

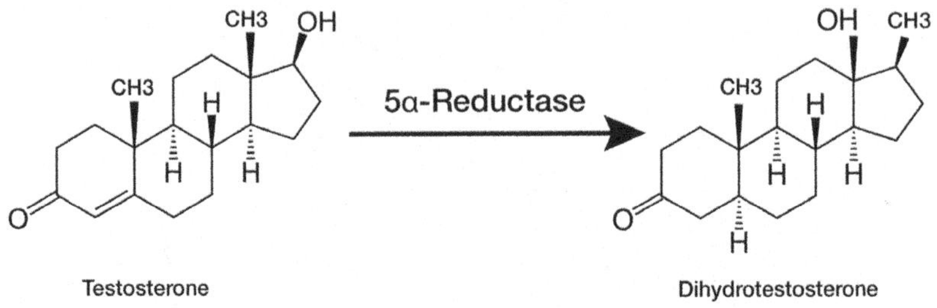

Diagram 32: Testosterone -> DHT (via 5-alpha reductase).

Certain products available for male pattern baldness and prostate enlargement work by blocking 5-alpha reductase (the enzyme that converts testosterone to DHT).

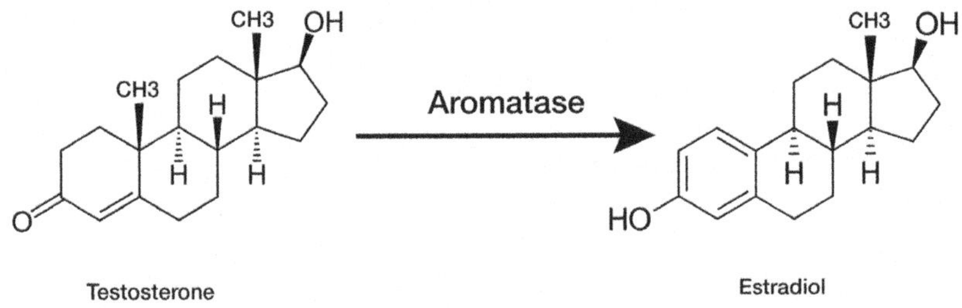

Diagram 33: Testosterone -> estradiol (via aromatase).

Testosterone and the Brain

Testosterone has multiple beneficial effects on the brain. It reduces anxiety and depression, and improves mood and memory.[191] Some of the antidepressant and antianxiety effects of testosterone come directly from testosterone. Others result after the conversion of testosterone to estradiol.

Because low testosterone is associated with cognitive decline, testosterone replacement improves cognitive functions and spatial abilities in men with low testosterone.[192] (Spatial abilities refers to the man's ability to make judgments about how he occupies space and perceives the space around him.)

Testosterone both indirectly (through the conversion to estradiol) and directly contributes to protection of nerve cells from stress that is due to free radicals (unstable atoms that can damage cells, causing illness and aging). The decline in circulating testosterone that comes with aging is related to an increased risk for neurodegenerative disorders.[193]

Testosterone and the Heart

Testosterone levels begin to decrease significantly after age forty, which has been associated with increased cardiovascular risk and all-cause mortality (death from all causes).

Low testosterone levels in men contribute to the risk of metabolic syndrome and type 2 diabetes, further increasing coronary artery disease risk.

Effects of testosterone on the heart

- Testosterone causes coronary artery dilation and increased blood flow in men with established coronary artery disease.
- The estrogen converted from testosterone has protective effects on blood vessel walls and prevents heart disease.
- Testosterone increases the functional capacity in men with heart failure.[194] This is likely due to testosterone's capability to generate energy in muscle cells, including heart muscle.
- Low testosterone levels in men with congestive heart failure are associated with a poor prognosis and increased mortality.[195, 196]
- Low testosterone levels are connected to increased risk of cardiovascular death.[197]

Studies showing cardiac benefits of testosterone therapy

A study showed that short-term intracoronary administration of testosterone at physiological (normal, healthy) doses caused coronary artery dilation, increasing coronary artery blood flow in men with established coronary artery disease.[198]

The authors of an article presented at the European Association of Urology (July 2022) reported that supplementing testosterone significantly reduces heart attacks and stroke in men who had naturally low levels of testosterone.

Testosterone replacement therapy improves:

- myocardial ischemia (reduced blood flow to the heart) in men with coronary artery disease,
- exercise capacity in patients with congestive heart failure,
- serum glucose levels,
- hemoglobin A1c (a long-term measure of blood sugar control), and
- insulin resistance in men with diabetes and prediabetes.

In men with heart failure and low testosterone levels, testosterone replacement therapy improved muscle sympathetic nerve activity, muscle wasting, and functional capacity.[199]

There can be severe effects on men when exercise reduces the blood flow in the heart (exercise-induced myocardial ischemia), including a heart attack. Researchers of three studies investigated this.

1. A study demonstrated that testosterone administration after exercise-induced myocardial ischemia in men with low testosterone levels produced a positive effect.[200]

2. Short-term testosterone administration had beneficial effects on exercise-induced myocardial ischemia in men

with coronary artery disease. This is thought to be due to direct, coronary-relaxing effects.[201]

3. Testosterone therapy has also been shown to reduce exercise-induced myocardial ischemia with men with chronic stable angina.[202]

Despite false claims about testosterone having negative effects on cardiovascular risk, there is no credible evidence that testosterone therapy *increases* cardiovascular risk, but there is substantial evidence that it does *not*.[203]

Insulin Sensitivity and the Metabolic Syndrome

Metabolic syndrome is a combination of disorders including insulin resistance, abnormal lipid profile, high blood pressure, excess abdominal fat, and increased risk for cardiovascular disease. It is a leading cause of mortality in aging men. Metabolic syndrome improves with testosterone replacement therapy, which has a positive effect on insulin sensitivity and insulin resistance.[204]

Testosterone therapy reduces obesity, fat mass, and waist circumference; improves blood sugar control; and reduces mortality.[205] Although testosterone replacement therapy is believed to *reduce* type 2 diabetes in men, it *increases* it in women.[206]

Long-term testosterone therapy improves components of metabolic syndrome and several inflammatory markers. The beneficial effects of testosterone therapy in men with type 2 diabetes include increasing insulin sensitivity, increasing lean mass, and decreasing subcutaneous fat.[207, 208]

Studies confirm that a newly-diagnosed metabolic syndrome can be reversed after fifty-two weeks of testosterone therapy in men with low testosterone.[209]

Testosterone and osteoporosis

Men with low testosterone have higher bone turnover and an increased risk of fractures. (Bone turnover is a natural process of replacing fragments of bone. It occurs throughout a person's life.) Treating these men with testosterone improves bone resorption; bone mass is maintained.

Testosterone's action on bone cells occurs directly via testosterone receptors as well as indirectly by first converting to estradiol via aromatase (an enzyme), which then attaches to the estrogen receptor on bone cells.

Studies confirm that estradiol contributes to the maintenance of bone mass after peak bone mass has been reached. Older men have low estradiol and an increased incidence of fractures.

Some men suffer from a mutation in their estrogen receptor gene or their aromatase enzyme (converts testosterone to estradiol) gene. These men have high bone turnover and low bone mass.[210]

Gonadal (from testes) and adrenal testosterone can be converted into estrogens by the P450 aromatase, which is present in many peripheral tissues, including bone. Bone can create (express) androgen receptors as well as estrogen receptors.

Skin

Testosterone has a beneficial effect on the skin—in healthy doses. It regulates epidermal skin moisture, elasticity, and skin thickness. Too much testosterone is linked to oily skin, clogged pores, and acne.

Muscle

Testosterone builds skeletal muscle through multiple mechanisms by improving muscle strength and power. Also, testosterone decreases fat while building lean body mass and improving body composition. Testosterone's effect on increasing the size of nerve cells facilitates the improvement in muscle strength and function.[211] Men of all ages benefit from this effect.

The muscle mass-building effects of testosterone led to abuse by athletes, which resulted in strict control of the distribution of testosterone. Therefore, athletes and bodybuilders misuse testosterone-like steroids (androgens) instead.

Neuroprotection

Testosterone plays a vital role in central nervous system development and has critical neuroprotective effects.[212] Testosterone prevents nerve cell death, improves memory after nerve damage, and regulates the activation and reactivity of glial cells (specialized supportive cells in the nervous system) after brain injury.

There is evidence that testosterone has protective effects in neurodegenerative disorders, such as Alzheimer's disease, mild cognitive impairment, and depression. Androgens affect the survival and regeneration of motor neurons. Researchers believe that testosterone replacement therapy may have a role in preventing and treating age-related disorders due to neuronal injury.[213]

The neuroprotective action of testosterone explains why the *decrease* in testosterone with aging is associated with an *increase* in neurodegenerative diseases. Other than the direct neuroprotective effects of testosterone, some of the benefits of testosterone occur after its conversion to estradiol and DHT.

Bone marrow stimulation

Testosterone stimulates the bone marrow to produce red blood cells. Testosterone therapy causes an *increase* in hemoglobin and hematocrit and a small decrease in HDL (high density lipids).[214]

The bone marrows of some men who receive replacement testosterone overproduce red blood cells. Therefore, healthcare providers need to order blood tests (hemoglobin and hematocrit) to monitor testosterone's effects on red blood cell production.

In some men, the stimulation of red blood cell production is very sensitive to testosterone. In this situation, healthcare providers must carefully regulate the testosterone dose. If hemoglobin increases too much when a man has normal, healthy blood testosterone levels, it is reasonable for him to donate blood every three to four months.

Strokes and TIAs

In older men, low testosterone levels have been associated with a higher incidence of stroke and TIAs (mini-strokes).[215]

Internal production of estradiol and testosterone in women and men is not associated with an increased risk of blood clots.[216] Physiological (healthy, normal levels) testosterone replacement does not adversely affect blood coagulation.[217]

Erectile and libido dysfunction

Through its effects on blood vessels and nerve tissue, testosterone contributes to the growth and function of penile tissue.

The most common cause of erectile dysfunction is limited blood flow in the penis. Reduced blood flow can be from:

- hardening arteries due to coronary artery disease,
- nerve damage from hyperglycemia and inadequately controlled blood glucose, or
- damage of arteries due to inadequate blood pressure.

Erectile dysfunction can also occur from stress, emotional issues, and prostate cancer.

Smoking can cause erectile dysfunction due to damage to blood vessels by the many harmful chemicals in tobacco smoke, which cause harm to arteries as well as many other organ systems. Also, nicotine reduces blood flow to the arteries.

Libido is the emotional interest in sex and is separate from erectile function. Often, erectile dysfunction and low libido have the same underlying cause: low testosterone.

Optimum testosterone levels are needed for vascular health, blood glucose control, and nerve health, which all contribute to the healthy blood vessels and nerves in the penile tissue. The damage to blood vessels and nerves resulting in erectile dysfunction commonly occurs sooner than the loss of libido, which is a psychological function.

Erectile dysfunction is more complex to resolve due to years of progressive changes and takes longer to improve. Healthy, normal ranges of testosterone will usually restore a healthy libido. A healthy lifestyle, long-term blood glucose control, and testosterone replacement therapy can improve erectile dysfunction over time.

Sperm production

Testosterone concentration in the testes must be 100 times more than blood levels for sperm development. Some of the testosterone produced in the testes is converted to estradiol, which is thought to help in sperm development. With testosterone replacement, the testes stop producing testosterone, and the sperm count plummets. However, this is not a reliable method of birth control.

Studies

Unfortunately, just as with estradiol and progesterone in women, minimal studies have been done on males receiving proper testosterone replacement. Most studies have been uncontrolled, observation studies with poor design, with the results manipulated using statistical analytic tools.

Taking study data and applying statistical analytical tools to achieve the desired outcome is a common but deceptive practice. One such study gained a lot of temporary attention from lawyers due to claiming testosterone replacement therapy increased the risk of stroke, myocardial infarction, and death. Review of the study showed that the results were the exact opposite but manipulated with statistical analytical tools.

Clinically, men who receive testosterone replacement in physiological doses report remarkable benefits. They specifically claim to have a better sleep, better cognition, better mood, better energy, better results with exercise on body composition, greater stamina, and better sexual function and libido.

12

PROSTATE CANCER, BPH, AND TESTOSTERONE

Prostate Cancer

The claim that testosterone replacement therapy *causes* prostate cancer is a medical myth created many years ago and *refuted* by several studies.

No studies have shown that testosterone therapy in men with low testosterone causes prostate cancer. According to several international guidelines, there is *no* conclusive evidence that testosterone therapy increases the risk of prostate cancer or BPH. There is also no evidence that testosterone treatment will convert subclinical (not causing symptoms) prostate cancer into clinically detectable prostate cancer.[218]

Men get prostate cancer well into andropause (age-related decline in testosterone), when their testosterone levels are low. In a study population of men who were treated with testosterone therapy for up to seventeen years, the incidence of prostate cancer was much lower than that reported in the general population of men who were not on testosterone therapy.[219]

Studies have repeatedly shown that prostate cancer is not caused by high testosterone levels. Testosterone replacement therapy for symptomatic men with low testosterone does not increase PSA (prostatic specific antigen, a substance that rises when a man has prostate cancer) levels, nor does it increase the risk of prostate cancer development.[220]

Like many other steroid hormones, testosterone stimulates cell growth, a critically important function. Hormones cannot discriminate between normal cells and malignant cells. If malignant cells have testosterone receptors, then they may take up testosterone just like normal cells do. There are numerous ways that malignant cells rapidly grow and spread. Malignant cells will grow and spread even if testosterone is not present, as testosterone is not what causes the malignancy.

Due to the lingering fear that malignant cells may take up testosterone, which can facilitate growth the same way that testosterone facilitates growth of normal cells, this hormone is not given to men with prostate cancer. Medications that block testosterone (anti-androgens), like Lupron, are usually given to slow prostate cancer, but they have not been shown to resolve it.

Studies concluded that testosterone use was not associated with aggressive prostate cancer and did not affect overall death due to cancer. Although study findings support growing evidence that testosterone replacement is safe for prostate cancer, more studies are needed to confirm this.[221]

BPH

BPH (benign prostatic hypertrophy) is a condition in aging men where the prostate gland enlarges. The urethra (the vessel transporting urine from the bladder to the penis) passes through the prostate gland. Urine flow is affected if the prostate gland enlarges and compresses the urethra.

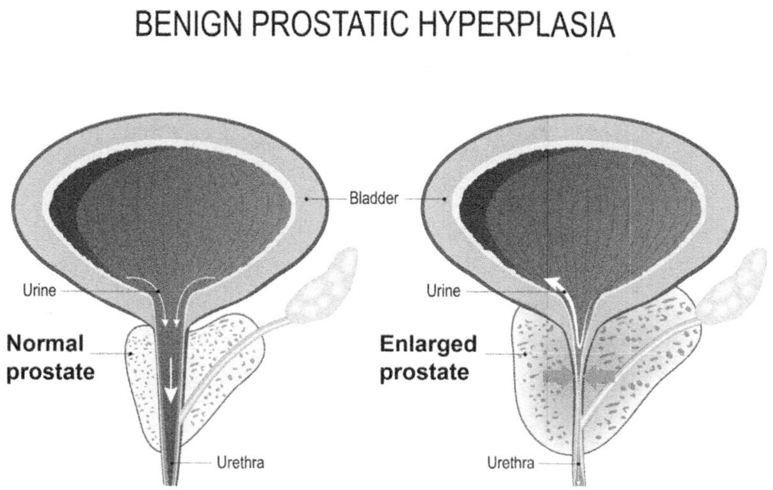

BENIGN PROSTATIC HYPERPLASIA

Diagram 34: BPH.

With age, testosterone levels decrease, and BPH increases. About 50 percent of men have BPH between fifty-one and sixty, and up to 90 percent have BPH after age eighty.

Although there is no consensus on why BPH develops, there are a few theories. BPH can likely develop due to several reasons, which is why some drugs work on some men, and other men require surgical treatment (since the same medications did not work on them).

The prostate gland comprises different tissue types (25 percent fibrous tissue, 25 percent muscular tissue, and 50 percent glandular tissue). Clinicians believe the front surface of the prostate (fibromuscular stroma) is stimulated by estrogen and inhibited by testosterone. The amount of testosterone and the testosterone to estradiol ratio declines with age. Some experts believe that the inner part of the prostate gland (stroma) enlarges due to the higher concentration of estradiol relative to testosterone, which expands the stroma and compresses the urethra. This enlargement causes BPH symptoms.

Other experts believe that BPH is due to varicoceles (the veins' enlargement that takes blood away from the testicle). All veins have valves that prevent backflow. Backflow occurs if the valves are damaged, which can happen with aging (such as in varicose veins).

According to a study published in the *Andrologia* medical journal in 2008,[222] age-related destruction of the valves in spermatic veins result in varicoceles. Elevated pressure within the varicocele diverts concentrated free testosterone directly from the testes to the prostate. The free testosterone then "feeds" the prostate gland, causing enlargement.

No study has shown testosterone replacement therapy to increase BPH, regardless of which theory is correct.

13

TESTOSTERONE IN WOMEN

In women, estradiol and progesterone are the primary sex steroids, but both women and men produce testosterone. Women make an average of fifteen to twenty times less testosterone than men.

Normal Testosterone Levels

For women in their fifties with balanced replacement of estradiol and progesterone, testosterone levels of thirty to forty ng/dL are reasonable. Younger women can naturally produce levels up to sixty ng/dL, but usually have much higher estradiol and progesterone levels. If they do not, they typically have excess facial hair or acne.

Where Is Testosterone Produced in Women?

The ovaries and adrenal glands make a small amount of testosterone. Before menopause, there is no precise data on how much testosterone in women comes from the adrenal glands versus the ovaries. Most likely, it varies individually.

After menopause, testosterone *only* comes from the adrenal glands. It results from the conversion of androstenedione (a weak adrenal hormone) and DHEA (dehydroepiandrosterone) to testosterone.

Benefits of Testosterone at Normal Levels in Women

Testosterone in women at normal female levels has several advantages, such as enhancing libido, improving sexual function, increasing metabolism, maintaining muscle mass, and increasing stamina.

Effects of Too Much Natural Production of Testosterone in Women

Women who naturally produce very high levels of testosterone are prone to health risks such as high blood pressure, high lipids, insulin resistance, and aggressive, hostile behavior. Physical attributes of too much testosterone include excess facial hair, acne, coarsening of facial features, changes in body composition, deepening of the voice, and frontal balding.

Risks of Abnormally High Testosterone Levels for Women

It is essential for women who are requesting testosterone replacement therapy to understand that higher than usual (supraphysiological) testosterone levels in females are associated with *metabolic syndrome*, including insulin resistance, hypertension, high cholesterol, and excess weight around the waist. Long-term, high-dose testosterone therapy in women can also eventually cause clitoromegaly (enlarged clitoris), male pattern baldness, facial hair, slight changes in facial muscles, voice changes, and other male characteristics, which are not all reversible.

Balance of Estradiol and Progesterone

Estradiol and progesterone are the primary female sex steroids with numerous beneficial effects on other hormones, including insulin and the cardiovascular system. When women receive testosterone replacement therapy, it is vital to keep estradiol, progesterone, and testosterone in balance and in physiological (normal, healthy) ranges.

Testosterone Replacement for Women to Enhance Libido

Women often take testosterone replacement to increase libido. If the woman's blood testosterone levels shifts into male ranges, the enhanced libido does not continue indefinitely, but the associated health risks do.

Taking testosterone replacement when adrenal glands are healthy may be a health risk. With healthy adrenal glands, replacing estradiol and progesterone in physiological (healthy, normal) doses will usually restore a healthy libido.

Testosterone Replacement for Bodybuilding

Bodybuilders often abuse testosterone and other synthetic anabolic steroids obtained through illegal sources. Although bodybuilders can achieve larger muscles, they expose themselves to significant health risks, as described previously.

Application Site

Application of testosterone cream or gel should be in non-fatty skin, as testosterone is fat-soluble and may linger in fatty tissue, converting to estrone and estradiol before being released into the bloodstream.

Baseline Testing and Monitoring

Before starting testosterone, it's advisable to get baseline fasting glucose levels and lipid profile, with follow-up levels being obtained a few times a year. The patient's medical records should include a few pre-testosterone therapy blood pressure readings, with close blood pressure monitoring during testosterone therapy.

14

BREAST CANCER

Breast cancer is one of the most feared diseases. It generates thoughts of painful treatment, disfigurement, loss of quality of life, and so much more.

Although rare, men can get breast cancer; this is a much more common disease in women. In women without a family history of breast cancer, the lifetime risk of breast cancer is about 13 percent, which means about 1 in 7.6 women will develop breast cancer in their life. Although we normally detect breast cancer earlier these days than we used to, survival for metastatic breast cancer (cancer that has spread beyond the local breast tissue) has not significantly changed. Overall survival remains at about 2.6 percent, with the five-year survival rate being about 29 percent (which means the chance of being alive with breast cancer in five years is 29 percent; however, that reduces to 2.6 percent for a normal life span).

For decades, the medical literature claimed that estrogen is linked to breast cancer. None of these claims have been substantiated or backed by any controlled studies. (See the section "Studies," later in this chapter, for more details on controlled studies and why their framework is critical.) Medical textbooks, books, and publications repeat these misleading claims of a connection between estrogen and breast cancer. This chapter will explore details surrounding the misconception and offer clarification based on facts that, for far too long, have mostly been overlooked.

How Does Cancer Start?

Cancer primarily results from uncorrected mutations of cells. Estradiol is a necessary hormone for women. It facilitates the normal growth and function of almost every cell in the body, including those in the breast, nervous system, bone, muscle, skin, and so on. If a mutation occurs in a previously normal breast cell with estradiol receptors, the mutant cell's growth may also be facilitated. The critical point is that estrogen did not *cause* cancer. (See the following section, "Estrogen Incorrectly Linked to Breast Cancer," for additional information.)

Breast cancer starts from *uncorrected* gene mutations. DNA mutations are an ongoing process, as is the body's constant surveillance and correction of these mutations. It is a fault in this repair system that can lead to cancer.

> **There are dozens of inherited gene mutations that increase the risk of breast cancer, the most common being BRCA 2 and BRCA 1. Other, less common ones include ATM gene, PAL B2, TP53, CHEK2, PTEN, CDH1, STK11, and LKB-1.**

Mutations can also occur from environmental factors such as radiation. Many other known and suspected carcinogens (substances that can trigger cancer) can overwhelm the body with mutations, hence leading to malignancy. Examples of a few carcinogens are benzene, asbestos, radon, vinyl chloride, nicotine, parabens, and tobacco smoke.

> **Patients with early exposure to ionizing radiation, especially for survivors of Hodgkin's lymphoma who received mantle radiation therapy, have a 25 percent increased lifetime risk of developing breast cancer.**

Estrogen Incorrectly Linked to Breast Cancer

Where did the idea arise that estrogen causes breast cancer and should be reduced or avoided? After all, estrogen is necessary for normal health and function. The misconception arose after pharmaceutical companies created synthetic (molecularly altered) versions of estrogen and turned them into pills mainly for hormone replacement therapy and contraception. These medications altered the natural balance and function of the body and created problems such as endometrial (uterine) cancer.

There was no increase in breast cancer seen when women received synthetic estrogen alone. To overcome the increased risk of endometrial cancer, pharmaceutical companies created synthetic *progesterone*, which proved to be harmful to the breast. The addition of synthetic progesterone to an estrogen-containing substance caused an increased risk of breast cancer. However, the false concept of a link between estrogen and breast cancer lingers.

It is well known that bioidentical progesterone in the natural cyclical regimen is safe and protective for the breast.[223] (See the following section, "Studies," for more details about the meaning of *bioidentical*.) Studies such as the Women's Health Initiative study confirmed the risk of breast cancer associated with synthetic progesterone.

Estrogen was used for decades without an increase in breast cancer.

Estrogen without progesterone caused an increased risk of endometrial (uterine) cancer.

Synthetic (fake) progesterone protects the uterus from endometrial cancer.

Synthetic (fake) progesterone does not protect the breast and is linked to breast cancer.

Real (bioidentical) progesterone is known to protect the breast, uterus and the rest of the body.[224]

To clarify the myth that estrogen increases the risk of breast cancer, consider three areas of evidence:

1. Studies,
2. What we historically observed, and
3. What we know from molecular studies.

Studies

There have been two types of studies on hormones in the past sixty years: uncontrolled and controlled studies. All kinds of studies are subject to misinterpretation and manipulation, mainly when statistical analytical tools are applied to the results to fabricate further desired outcomes and obscure the proper conclusions.

The following information applies to studies of *bioidentical hormones* about hormone replacement therapy. *To date, no medical study* has used completely bioidentical hormones in a safe route of administration or in physiological (normal human) doses.

Bioidentical is a term that refers to the molecular structure of a molecule, and it essentially means that the exact atomic composition of the molecule is identical to what the human body makes. For health, this makes all the difference.

Uncontrolled studies

An uncontrolled study is the weakest type of study and subject to the most errors. The participants self-report the data collected (over the years), then it is analyzed and presented. The study group is not compared to anyone else or placebo.

The **Million Women Study** from the UK and the **Nurses' Health Study** from the US are the two major uncontrolled studies. Both showed a slight increase in breast cancer in the women who reported using postmenopausal hormone replacement therapy, especially those using combined synthetic estrogen and synthetic progesterone.

These studies were heavily criticized and refuted due to several reasons, including poor design and data interpretation. The damage that they caused still lingers in the minds of many healthcare providers. The notion that estrogen is linked to breast cancer mainly stemmed from these studies, evidenced by the multitude of publications and literature referring back to these studies as being a source of authority. Human progesterone protects the breast as well as endometrial tissue from cancer development. Researchers never focused on the role of synthetic progesterone because, at the time, doctors did not know (and most still don't know) the difference between synthetic and real (human) progesterone.

Controlled studies

Controlled studies are the most robust and most reliable studies. Here, the participants are more carefully selected, usually put into randomly assigned groups to receive either a placebo (sugar pill) or the active drug being tested, and they are closely followed by a team of investigators.

The patients taking a placebo do not know they are not receiving an active medication. This makes it a "blind" study. In some cases, the researchers do not know which subjects received the placebo until the study is over. (This is called a double-blind study, meaning both the patients and researchers are both in the dark.) Patients who participate in these studies sign an extensive informed consent before starting and know that they might receive either a placebo or the active medication.

The Women's Health Initiative study is the most significant study to date. It shook the world of hormone replacement therapy and made hormone therapy more controversial than ever. The study's design and the presentation of results were careless and damaging. The results were prematurely reported and incorrectly interpreted.

- The study only used synthetic hormones
- Patients received oral estrogen, known to be a risk for blood clots.
- The results did not clarify that *synthetic progesterone* was linked to **increased** breast cancer.
- The researchers did not stress that *estrogen* was linked to **less** breast cancer.

The **Danish Osteoporosis Prevention Study** was initiated in 1990 and ended in 1993, involving 1006 women.

- Participants received bioidentical estradiol and synthetic progesterone.
- The women who used estradiol (estrogen) alone had significantly **reduced breast cancer**.

The **KEEPS (Kronos Early Estrogen Prevention Study)** is the latest study to date. It began in 2005, shortly after the Women's Health Initiative study ended in 2004.

- Participants received either synthetic estrogen or transdermal (applied to the skin) bioidentical estradiol with oral bioidentical progesterone.
- **The results showed no increase in breast cancer.**

Historical Observations

Early menarche and late menopause

Some healthcare providers incorrectly believe that women who had an early menarche (start of period) and late menopause have more breast cancer, which is allegedly due to more exposure to estrogen. This conclusion is an example of incomplete information resulting in regurgitated nonsense. There is no solid data to support this.

Suppose that early menarche and late menopause were linked to increased risk of breast cancer. In that case, this connection could be due to many other hormonal imbalances or genetic factors and not just erroneously assumed it's due to estrogen. If hormone imbalance has a risk of breast cancer, it could be due to the low progesterone state of both early menarche and late menopause. Low progesterone could be a significant factor linked to breast cancer.[225]

High estrogen states

In various books and journal articles, authors falsely state that high estrogen states are linked to breast cancer. Clinically, we see the *opposite*.

- Pregnancy is a known **high** estrogen state; however, women with more pregnancies have **less** breast cancer.

- Nulliparity (no pregnancies) is a **low** estrogen state and is linked to a **higher** risk of breast cancer.

- Increasing age is a **low** estrogen state and is linked to a **higher** risk of breast cancer; breast cancer rates increase after menopause.

- Use of birth control pills, which induces a very **low** estrogen state, along with synthetic progesterone, is linked to a **high** risk of breast cancer.

- Implementation of IUDs, especially with synthetic progesterone, is associated with a **low** estrogen state and linked to **increased** breast cancer.

Breast cancer is seen **less often** in high estrogen states, examples of such include an increased number of pregnancies and youth.

Breast cancer is seen **more often** in low estrogen states, examples of such include use of birth control pills, implementation of IUDs, and older age.

Molecular Studies

Some drug companies have taken an active interest in molecular studies designed to test theories about estrogen. A few groups of researchers are determined to prove that the estrogen in a woman's body is a risk for initiating breast cancer. This position allows justification for introducing a drug that clears the estrogen in a woman's body:

1. After menopause, the ovaries no longer make estrogen. A small amount of estrogen continues to be made indirectly from the adrenal glands.

2. The adrenal glands in healthy women make testosterone, some of which converts to estrogen. Although this is a small amount of estrogen, it is valuable.

3. By "proving" that estrogen causes breast cancer, pharmaceutical companies want to sell a drug that stops the conversion of testosterone to estrogen as a solution to reduce the risk of breast cancer after menopause. A fundamental issue with that idea is the reality that estradiol is an important hormone with countless benefits, including providing immune protection. Removing it from the body is not a safe thing to do.

This goal is an alarming scheme by pharmaceutical giants to promote a deceptive use of a drug that may have some temporary benefit in limiting local tumor growth in metastatic breast cancer.

Big Pharma is trying to promote the use of their medications to prevent breast cancer when there is absolutely no evidence that estradiol causes breast cancer.

Researchers subjected genetically altered mice to high estrogen levels without also subjecting them to additional progesterone (a scenario that does not occur in healthy animals). The goal is to try to prove estrogen causes breast cancer. By creating some scenario where it may seem estrogen is causing breast cancer (even if it is an artificial, unnatural environment), it can give drug companies a reason to promote aromatase inhibitors (AIs) drugs, which reduce the conversion of testosterone to estrogen, as a solution to prevent breast cancer in postmenopausal women with a family history of breast cancer. The family history of breast cancer is due to mutations in cancer surveillance genes, not an adverse reaction to estrogen.

No studies have shown a mechanism proving that estrogen initiates or increases the risk of breast cancer.

Mutations in Breast Cancer

It is critical to recognize that there is not a connection between estrogen and mutations. Once a breast cell mutates and escapes the normal mutation surveillance, it rapidly multiplies. Estrogen may or may not facilitate the growth of those cells the way that it does normal cells.

Malignant cells lose control of their rate of growth and boundaries. They leave their normal environment, enter the lymphatic system, and metastasize (spread). This is a devastating event. Neither the mutation nor metastasis was caused by estrogen.

When cancer is only in the breast, surgery often cures the patient. Chemotherapy prolongs survival for patients with metastatic disease. If a tumor is large and causing pain, such as impinging on the spine, drugs that stop estrogen production may provide some temporary relief (but not a cure) by temporarily limiting or shrinking the growth, but they are not destroying the tumor or stopping its spread. Estrogen can never be completely removed from the body. Unfortunately, it is rarely possible to kill all metastasized cancer cells. It is important to understand that estrogen does not cause cancer. If a cell has estrogen receptors, estrogen will enter that cell and cause growth the way that it does everywhere else in non-cancerous cells. But again, the estrogen is **not the cause** of the cancer, it is merely interacting with the cancer cells that already exist.

For certain patients, there may be a small temporary benefit to receiving aromatase inhibitors (AIs) for metastatic breast cancer treatment. If breast cancer cells have estrogen receptors, then depriving them of estrogen will locally slow their growth. Unfortunately, this is not a cure, and does not stop the spread of cancer.

Hormone Replacement in Women with a History of Breast Cancer

Whether to take hormone replacement when a woman has had breast cancer is a dilemma. It warrants a thorough, unbiased investigation. Estrogen and progesterone are necessary for health and well-being. Studies have shown that estrogen therapy after a history of breast cancer does *not* increase the chance of recurrent or new cancer, but further clarification is needed. The greatest hindrance to success is drug companies pushing drugs promising to deplete a woman's estrogen and reduce the risk of breast cancer.

In the 1990s, researchers completed a study on 319 women previously treated for breast cancer. The women received estrogen replacement therapy to see how it affected the development of new or recurrent breast cancer. The results, published in the *Journal of Clinical Oncology* in 1999, showed that estrogen replacement therapy did not increase breast cancer events.[226]

A follow-up study showed that estrogen replacement therapy did not compromise disease-free survival in patients previously for localized breast carcinoma. Results were published in the *Cancer* journal in 2002.[227]

The *Annals of Surgical Oncology* from 2001 reported a study done on 607 breast cancer survivors regarding the use of estrogen replacement. Researchers followed sixty-four patients and found that fifty-six reported receiving some sort of estrogen replacement therapy after the breast cancer diagnosis. Seventy-four percent of those patients previously had estrogen-positive tumors. The twelve-year study showed that estrogen replacement therapy was *not* associated with increased breast cancer events compared to non-estrogen replacement therapy uses.[228]

Summary

- No study to date has shown that any type of estrogen causes breast cancer.

- The **Women's Health Initiative study** showed that synthetic (fake) progesterone is linked to breast cancer. We know that our own (bioidentical) progesterone is protective to every part of our body, including the breast. The study also showed that women who took estrogen without the synthetic progesterone had less breast cancer.

- Birth control pills and hormone replacement therapy used in the **Nurses' Health Study** and **Million Women's Study** showed a slight increase in breast cancer. Blood levels of estradiol in women using oral hormone replacement therapy or birth control pills is very low (menopausal levels). Those women also used synthetic progesterone, which is linked to breast cancer.

- Although estrogen does NOT cause breast cancer, estrogen is a steroid hormone that causes growth of tissue. If a malignant breast cancer cell has estrogen receptors, estrogen will enter it. If it is a local growth, the tumor will locally grow and likely be detected early and removed. Once breast cancer spreads beyond the breast, the only time estrogen deprivation can temporarily help is by slowing the growth of a large tumor that is causing pain and is not amenable to resection or radiation therapy. But the success of this is limited and temporary. Estrogen deprivation is not a cure.

15

THYROID GLAND

Normal levels of thyroid hormone are necessary for every aspect of health, including normal growth and development. At different developmental stages, the thyroid hormone serves different functions. The fetus cannot develop properly without adequate thyroid hormone and depends on the mother to have normal thyroid hormone levels.

Unlike gonadal hormones (estradiol, progesterone, and testosterone), a deficiency in thyroid hormone is considered a medical disease and addressed by mainstream medicine, although usually not in an optimal way.

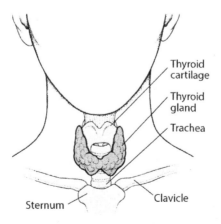

Diagram 35: Thyroid gland.

Thyroid hormone is produced by the thyroid gland, which is located in the front of the mid-neck area. It has a strong blood supply and extensive nerve connections.

Thyroid hormone production is controlled by the hypothalamus and the pituitary gland, which are hormone-producing glands in the brain. Through a complex feedback loop, the hypothalamus releases Thyroid Releasing Hormone (TRH), which triggers the pituitary gland to release Thyroid Stimulating Hormone (TSH). TSH stimulates the thyroid gland to release T4 and T3.

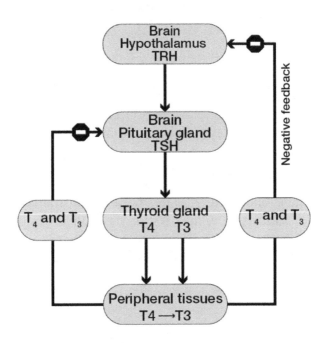

Diagram 36: Feedback loop.

Types of Thyroid Hormone

There are four different types of thyroid hormone (T4, T3, T2, and T1), each identified by the number and position of iodine atoms.

About 90 percent of the thyroid hormone exists as T4, and about 9 percent exists as T3. A small portion exists as an inactive form of T3, called reverse T3.

T4 (Thyroxine)

The main thyroid hormone is T4 (also known as thyroxine) and is the storage form of thyroid hormone. T4 is stored in the thyroid gland as well as several other parts of the body, including the liver and kidneys.

T3 (Triiodothyronine)

T3 is the active form of thyroid hormone. It is converted from T4 by countless known and unknown factors. We know that the levels of the active thyroid hormone (T3) varies during the day. T3 levels are typically higher in the morning. Due to the interaction of ovarian hormones (especially estradiol) with thyroid function, there is a variation in T3 production during the ovarian cycle. Interestingly, men seem to have fewer thyroid deficiency complaints than women.

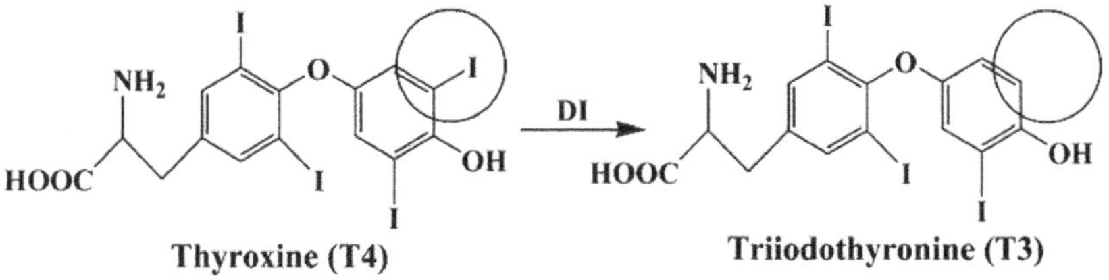

Diagram 37: Conversion of T4 to T3 (via deiodinase).

The Thyroid Gland with Aging

Thyroid hormone production and efficiency diminishes with aging. As individuals move further down away from their personal healthy ranges of thyroid hormone, symptoms of hypothyroidism develop, eventually leading to dysfunction and imbalance in other hormone systems. (See "Symptoms and Effects of Hypothyroidism," later in this chapter, for more information.)

Functions of Thyroid Hormone

Normal thyroid function is critical for balanced health. Too low or too high levels of thyroid hormone is a medical emergency.

Thyroid hormone affects every aspect of well-being and is connected to every other hormone system in the body, including an intricate connection to insulin, estradiol, and other steroid hormones. As mentioned previously, an imbalance in the thyroid system ultimately affects other important functions in the body.

A Few Other Important Actions of Thyroid Hormone

- Every organ system including the heart, liver, and kidneys are dependent on thyroid balance.[229, 230, 231, 232, 233, 234]

- Thyroid hormone regulates cell function and basic metabolic rate.

- Energy production (via the cell mitochondria) involves thyroid hormone.[235, 236, 237]

- Thyroid hormone is involved in regulating lipid balance, affecting levels of triglycerides, cholesterol, and LDL receptors.[238]

- Thyroid hormone is involved in fat synthesis and breakdown as well as protein turnover.

- Thyroid hormone plays an important role in normal brain and nervous system development, maturation, and function, including nerve cell generation, cognition, and mood balance.[239, 240, 241, 242]

- Thyroid hormones help with healthy scalp hair and hair pigmentation.
- Thyroid hormone contributes to balancing skin function, including moisture and skin pigmentation.
- Thyroid hormone has a direct effect on muscle movement (which is why we test reflexes for thyroid function).

Symptoms and Effects of Hypothyroidism

Cold intolerance, constipation, physical fatigue, weight gain, slow metabolic rate, mental slowness, excessive sleepiness, depression, thinning hair, thinning eyebrows, slow speech, hoarse voice, prolonged reflexes, cardiac dysfunction, ovarian dysfunction, insulin resistance, are some of the symptoms associated with hypothyroidism.

Some of the Causes of Hypothyroidism

Hashimoto's disease is an autoimmune disorder, and it is the most common cause of hypothyroidism. Other than age-related decline in thyroid function, hypothyroidism can also be caused by inflammatory conditions including viral illnesses, cancer, radiation exposure, medications, iodine deficiency, or too much iodine (Wolff-Chaikoff effect).

More recently, during the COVID-19 pandemic, it was observed that subacute thyroiditis (immune reaction of the thyroid gland) increased in patients after being diagnosed with COVID-19.[243]

Lab Testing for Thyroid Function

Most women suffer for years without treatment because they are still within the "normal" range of standard lab testing. As with most hormone levels, the "normal" range that labs use is an average for the population and does not adjust for the individual's personal optimal range.

Currently, standard-of-care medicine does not typically treat an under-functioning thyroid gland unless the TSH and T4 values are outside the "normal" lab range.

Women who have symptoms of an under-functioning thyroid gland often have normal T4 and TSH levels but have T3 values that are borderline low to below normal, due to some defect in conversion of T4 to T3, which is not completely understood. Most physicians still only check TSH and occasionally T4. In many cases, this is not adequate. **TSH**, **Free T3**, and **Free T4** levels (not just T3 and T4) must be checked in anyone who complains of symptoms consistent with hypothyroidism. In more rare cases, T4 converts to reverse T3, which is an inactive form of T3.

Treating Hypothyroidism

Although the most common cause of hypothyroidism is Hashimoto's disease, thyroid gland function commonly decreases with aging. Before treating hypothyroidism, it is important to have a medical evaluation to rule out other metabolic deficiencies or medical conditions.

Giving thyroid replacement with an underlying adrenal insufficiency can be dangerous, and the adrenal deficiency needs to be treated first. Individuals with cardiac dysfunction should also be closely monitored.

Synthroid and its generic versions, including Levothyroxine, is T4 and is the standard medical treatment for low thyroid function. This can be a good choice if the body is converting adequate amounts of T4 to T3, which can be monitored by routine blood tests.

Armour Thyroid is derived and prepared from pig tissue. It consists of T4, T3, T2, and T1. Over the last ten years, Armour Thyroid has gained increased acceptance in the medical community, however, endocrinologists are still hesitant in prescribing this vs. standard therapy with T4. Other preparations of thyroid hormone also exist, but not much data is available on them.

Some women prefer to use a T4 preparation with a small dose of a commercial T3 preparation (Cytomel, also known as Liothyronine). Anyone on thyroid hormone replacement should be routinely monitored by blood tests, and for symptoms.

Hyperthyroidism (Overactive Thyroid Function)

Excess thyroid hormone is usually due to overstimulation of the thyroid gland. The most common disease associated with hyperthyroidism is Graves's disease, which is an autoimmune disease with some genetic predisposition.

Too much thyroid hormone causes symptoms such as an increase in heart rate, excess sweating, heat intolerance, tremor, palpitations, tiredness, fatigue, nervousness, skin changes, eye problems including bulging eyes, and increase in appetite.

Extremely high levels of thyroid hormone is a medical emergency. Hyperthyroidism involves treatment that requires close monitoring by an endocrinologist.

16

ADRENAL GLANDS

We have two adrenal glands, which are located above the kidneys. The adrenal glands are essential for sustaining life, regulating metabolism, adapting to stress, and countless other critical functions.

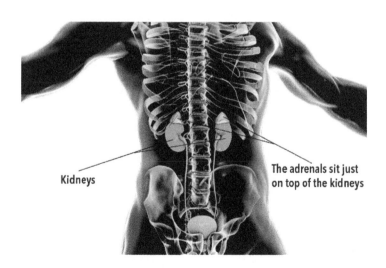

Kidneys

The adrenals sit just on top of the kidneys

Diagram 38: Position of the adrenal glands.

We need healthy adrenal glands throughout our lives. Diseases of the adrenal glands, such as Cushing syndrome, Addison's disease, and several congenital disorders, need lifelong treatment and close monitoring.

The adrenal gland is incredibly complex. It directly communicates with the brain hormones and chemicals, the gonads (ovaries and testes), and every other organ, neurotransmitter, and hormone in the body. The brain and the adrenal glands are the most complex hormone-producing structures in the body. Although we know a lot about the adrenal gland function, there is so much more that we do not know.

Like the brain, the adrenal glands can get stressed due to constant physical and mental fatigue. However, unless there is a functional defect in the brain or adrenal hormone production, the adrenal glands can recover from fatigue with behavioral changes rather than supplements and medications. Healthcare practitioners should use great caution and judgment before prescribing anything that can alter the natural internal balance of the adrenal glands or the brain.

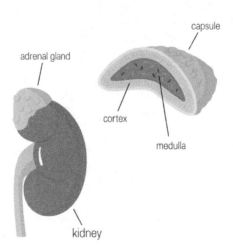

ADRENAL GLAND

Diagram 39

Adrenal glands overwork and undergo additional stress after per-imenopause, menopause, and andropause due to compensating for normal gonadal hormone levels. If estradiol and progesterone in women and testosterone in men are correctly replaced, the adrenal glands can generally recover.

Adrenal Medulla

The inner part of the adrenal gland, the medulla, produces cate-cholamines, such as norepinephrine and epinephrine (adrenaline). Catecholamines are categorized as hormones and function as neurotransmitters (communicate through nerve endings).

Catecholamines engage in the body's "fight-or-flight" response and are released in response to high stress and fear. They increase blood glucose levels and increase heart rate and cardiac out-put while controlling blood flow in other organs to facilitate the fight-or-flight response.

Adrenal Cortex

The outer part of the adrenal gland is the cortex, and it produces steroid hormones. The cells of the adrenal cortex have numerous receptors for cholesterol. Every steroid hormone is derived from cholesterol.

The adrenal cortex has three layers:

1. **The outer layer** makes aldosterone. Its main job is to reg-ulate salt and water balance via the kidneys.
2. **The middle layer** makes cortisol, which has numerous life-sustaining functions. It is the primary stress hormone and controls inflammation and suppresses immune reactions.
3. **The inner layer** makes androgens, which consist of DHEA and androstenedione, which convert to testosterone, DHT, and estrogens outside the adrenal glands.

Regulation of Adrenal Steroid Hormones

The steroid hormones of the adrenal gland are tightly regulated in a complex process involving the brain hormones Corticotropin Releasing Hormone (CRH) and Adrenocorticotropic Hormone (ACTH), as well as multiple other factors which are not as well understood.

Adrenal Androgens

Adrenarche is a developmental change regulated by the adrenal glands. It shows up as the growth of axillary and pubic hair, production of sweat glands, skin changes, and changes in sexual characteristics. Adrenarche occurs before puberty and the onset of the menstrual cycle (menarche).

The adrenal glands make dehydroepiandrosterone (DHEA), dehydroepiandrosterone sulfate (DHEAS), and androstenedione. These hormones change to testosterone, DHT, estrone, and estradiol outside the adrenal glands. DHEA gets broken down after about fifteen to thirty minutes and is therefore converted to DHEAS, which lasts longer (seven to ten hours).

DHEA and DHEAS steadily peak until the mid-twenties, then start to decline with age.[244] There is a linear decline of DHEA in both men and women of about 2 percent a year, starting at age thirty. The decline is more prominent in women than men and is thought to be due to the decline in estradiol.[245]

There is a definite but unclear relationship between ovarian hormones and adrenal testosterone production. Ovaries typically produce a baseline level of testosterone. However, after the mid-menstrual cycle peak and drop in estradiol just before ovulation, there is a sharp rise in testosterone. This rise may come from the adrenal glands and increases libido. Once estrogen and progesterone rise again, the testosterone levels trend down to baseline.

Women who are under stress have a lower libido and difficulty conceiving. It is challenging to restore a healthy libido if adrenal glands remain under stress.

During late perimenopause and menopause, some women develop acne, chin hair, and hair loss with central balding. These hair changes are due to the adrenal gland compensation by making DHEA, which converts to testosterone (acne and chin hair), which further converts to DHT (central balding) without the balancing effects of progesterone and estradiol.

This adrenal compensation does not happen to everyone, nor does it always last very long, as, after a while, the adrenal glands "burn out."

Regulation of DHEA and DHEAS

We know very little about the regulation of DHEA and DHEAS. There appears to be an increase in DHEA production with the increase of the brain hormones CRH and ACTH, which is why it is important to be cautious when taking adrenal supplements.

To date, no trial or study has demonstrated the long-term safety of DHEA replacement. Studies have shown that oral DHEA administration in women with hypoadrenal function results in unfavorable lipid levels. This change is likely because DHEA converts to testosterone, and it is well known that testosterone negatively affects lipid profile in women.

Studies have shown that women who had androgen deficiency due to pituitary dysfunction and received supplemental testosterone initially felt benefits, such as psychological well-being, improved sexual function, improved bone mineral density, and lean body mass. However, long-term data is not available.

In women with adrenal insufficiency due to pituitary dysfunction, ovarian hormones should be balanced with adrenal hormones, and the ratio of testosterone to estradiol and progesterone levels must be within the normal ranges. Women with low estradiol and progesterone and high androgens (such as testosterone, DHT, and DHEA) are at risk for metabolic syndrome.

17

GROWTH HORMONE

Human growth hormone (HGH) is a protein hormone made in the brain's pituitary gland and released in a pulsatile manner. (*Pulsatile* means released in spurts.) It is necessary for the correct growth, development, and maintenance of health.

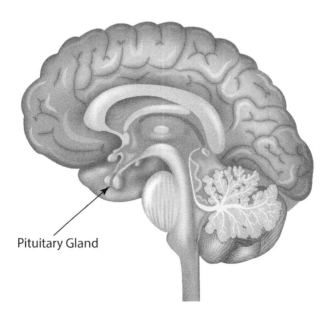

Pituitary Gland

Diagram 40

Growth Hormone in Children

In children, growth hormone is necessary for proper growth and development of the body. Children who have insufficient growth hormone or have growth hormone resistance experience stunted growth or dwarfism.

Too much growth hormone in children during the growth phase results in gigantism (acromegaly). If untreated, a child could be as tall as eight feet or more.

Growth Hormone in Adults

In adults, a balance of growth hormone is necessary for the proper functioning of the body.[246] Growth hormone production slows down after about age thirty by approximately 15 percent every decade.

Unfortunately, some athletes take the growth hormone to achieve better performance. Also, some prescribers overtreat patients without following proper guidelines. Therefore, FDA approval of growth hormone is very limited, and its use is illegal for "anti-aging" or bodybuilding purposes.

Overtreatment with growth hormone results in excessive growth of certain flat bones. This excess most often affects the bones of the face, skull, hands, feet, and so on. Too much growth hormone can also cause excessive poor-quality muscle development, insulin resistance, lipid disorders, nerve problems, carpal tunnel syndrome, and other metabolic derangements.

Our natural growth hormone decreases with age and affects different individuals differently. Although treatment with growth hormone for "anti-aging" purposes is illegal, growth hormone can significantly increase the quality of life in certain individuals who are already optimized in other hormone systems (thyroid, adrenal, gonadal).

Growth Hormone Replacement

Growth hormone treatment has benefits in several situations where other treatments have been unsuccessful.

- Low growth hormone levels result in a low quality of life, including altered body composition with reduced muscle mass, excess fat, and excessive fatigue, among other symptoms.[247]

- Growth hormone reduces insulin resistance in obese individuals with functional growth hormone deficiency.[248, 249]

- Certain drug-resistant seizure disorders show improvement with growth hormone treatment.[250]

- Studies of individuals with growth hormone deficiency, memory, mood, psychological well-being, self-esteem, and mental fatigue showed improvement with growth hormone treatment.[251, 252]

- Studies have shown that testosterone's effect on improving body composition in older men was enhanced by growth hormone supplementation.[253, 254, 255, 256]

- Patients with chronic pain, fibromyalgia, and fatigue have been shown to benefit from growth hormone therapy.[257]

- Growth hormone has a vital role in the regeneration of tissue growth and maintenance, including survival of special retinal nerve cells.[258]

- The thymus gland, which has immune-related functions in adults, relies on the growth hormone for normal maintenance.[259]

Normal growth hormone levels in adults increase lean body mass and fat loss, improve lipid profile, and play an essential role in regulating cell function and division.

Oxidative stress is a term that reflects a damaging environment in the cell. Chemical reactions are constantly taking place,

producing highly charged, bullet-like molecules called free radicals as byproducts. Small amounts of free radicals are necessary
to ignite further essential cell reactions, and the damage by free
radicals is usually taken care of by the cells in our damage repair
system. Over time, there is more damage than repair, resulting in
oxidative stress. Growth hormone and insulin-like growth factors
balance free radicals and curtail oxidative stress.

Many factors affect the pulsatile secretion of growth hormone,
including estradiol and testosterone levels, exercise, age, and
body composition.[260, 261, 262, 263, 264] Growth hormone is a protein hormone and requires cell receptors to enter the cell. Estrogen works
with the growth hormone secretion to increase cell receptors for
growth hormone. Administering growth hormone without first
replacing estrogen in women and testosterone in men does not
give an optimal result.

Measuring Growth Hormone Levels

Growth hormone has a brief duration and gets broken down
quickly. Also, the pulsatile nature of release makes getting an
accurate measurement challenging. However, growth hormone
directly stimulates the release of insulin-like growth factor (IGF-1)
from the liver, which exists at a more constant level in the blood.
Therefore, IGF-1 levels are often used as an indicator of growth
hormone status.[265, 266]

The standard medical test to measure growth hormone deficiency
due to low production from the pituitary gland is the Growth
Hormone Stimulation Test. The test involves measuring blood
over two to five hours before and after injecting a growth hormone
stimulant (usually a particular amino acid). Because the levels of
growth hormone decrease by about 15 percent every decade, and
the "normal" levels from the lab are reduced for increasing age,
it's possible to have low functional levels of growth hormone but
not a low level on the lab report.

Proper Use of Growth Hormone

As mentioned above, growth hormone is tightly regulated and cannot be used off-label (for a use other than approved by the FDA). The FDA banned the use of growth hormone for any use other than a documented deficiency in the production and release of growth hormone from the pituitary gland in the brain. Unfortunately, the measurements required for evaluating the release of growth hormone from the pituitary gland and the criteria for deficiency are outdated and insufficient. They do not take into consideration the age-related decline.

Growth hormone is extracted from animal brain tissue. It should never be obtained from any facility that is not FDA approved, especially if the formulation is injectable. If the proper extraction and purification is not done, there is a risk of transmitting fatal brain disease.

Growth hormone should not be replaced before the adrenals, thyroid glands, and gonadal hormones (estradiol, progesterone, and testosterone) are within normal range. Replacing growth hormone with underlying developing adrenal insufficiency or low thyroid hormone levels (hypothyroidism) can worsen symptoms. This is not a hormone that can be used without the utmost caution and close monitoring. Although there are sources on the internet of growth hormone, patients should never purchase this for unsupervised use. The structural changes in the body, including bone changes, that occur with excess growth hormone are irreversible. A well-informed physician should guide the use of the medication to ensure that the dose is within a safe range.

CONCLUSION

Estradiol and progesterone in women and testosterone in men are essential for our health and well-being. It is the decline and loss of these hormones that result in the rapid aging and senile degeneration. Replacing in normal, human ranges (physiological ranges) the exact hormones that our bodies made is one of the most powerful steps in remaining healthy, vibrant, and youthful for the rest of our lives.

Our healthcare system is heavily influenced by Big Pharma, who—as part of the medical industry—are primarily sustained by treating chronic, age-related diseases. Hormone replacement has only recently been accepted by mainstream medicine as an option for addressing menopausal symptoms, however, hormone replacement for the prevention of chronic diseases is still meeting resistance.

As early as the 1930s, Fuller Albright, a renowned scientist and endocrinologist, identified that the loss of estradiol resulted in osteoporosis. Thousands of scientific studies thereafter have clearly shown the health benefits of estradiol and progesterone in women and testosterone in men for every aspect of health. No well-designed study to date has been conducted using the hormones the human body makes (bioidentical) in physiological doses.

Estradiol has such profound health benefits that men will naturally convert a portion of testosterone to estradiol to achieve estradiol's critical health benefits. No human study has proved that estradiol is linked to breast cancer. Only fake (synthetic) progesterone has been shown to increase the risk of breast cancer. It is important to understand the facts, so that the decision on hormone replacement therapy is not based on false information.

The debilitating effects of senile degeneration are felt more significantly from our seventies and onwards, when the effects of mental decline and degeneration of the musculoskeletal system continue to take away our quality of life and independence. When deciding on what course to take regarding the aging process, it is important to understand the scientific facts, and not rely on ill-informed healthcare providers or the abundant amount of misinformation that floods the internet, mainly provided by entities whose financial interests conflict with our best interests.

After our fifties, we should enjoy life the most. Our brain and mental function should be strong and healthy. Rather than mentally slowing down, we should draw from our rich life experiences and knowledge to enjoy a higher level of intellectual function that is not possible without the experience factor. We should not have to suffer from the degeneration of our muscles, bones, ligaments, tendons, or joints, but instead we should be able to live in dignity and strength.

REVIEW INQUIRY

I hope you've enjoyed the book, finding it both useful and informative. I believe that the information in this book is vital for everyone to be aware of, and I hope to make it available to the many women and men who are aging without knowing their options. Your input would be very helpful.

Would you consider giving it a rating wherever you bought the book? Online book stores are more likely to promote a subject when they feel good about its content, and reader reviews are a great barometer for a book's quality.

So please go to the website of wherever you bought the book, search for my name and the book title, and leave a review. If able, perhaps consider adding a picture of you holding the book. That increases the likelihood your review will be accepted!

Many thanks in advance,

Selma Rashid, MD

Get this book for a friend, associate, or family member!

If you have found this book valuable and know others who would find it useful, consider buying them a copy as a gift. Special bulk discounts are available if you would like your whole team or organization to benefit from reading this. Just contact DrSelmaRashid@gmail.com or visit AntiAgingMedicalGroup.com.

Would You Like Dr. Selma to Speak to Your Organization?

Book Selma now!

Dr. Selma Rashid accepts a limited number of speaking engagements each year. To learn how you can bring her message to your organization, email DrSelmaRashid@gmail.com or visit AntiAgingMedicalGroup.com.

ENDNOTES

Introduction

1. Manson, J. E., R. T. Chlebowski, and R. B. Wallace. "The Women's Health Initiative Hormone Therapy Trails: Update and Overview of Health Outcomes During the Intervention and Post-Stopping Phases." *JAMA* 310(13) (Oct 2, 2013): 1353–1368.

Chapter 1: Controversies About Hormone Replacement Therapy

2. Kling, J. "The Strange Case of Premarin Modern Drug Discovery." *Modern Day Discovery.* ASC Publications. 3(8) (2000): 46–52. Available at: http://pubs.acs.org/subscribe/archive/mdd/v03/i08/html/kling.html. Accessed July 22, 2019.

3. Wilson, Robert A. "The Role of Estrogen and Progesterone in Breast and Genital Cancer." *JAMA* 182(4) (1962): 327–331. DOI: 10.1001/jama.1962.03050430001001.

4. Ziel, H. K., and W. D. Finkle. "Increased risk of endometrial carcinoma among users of conjugated estrogens." *N. Engl. J. Med.* 293 (1975): 1167–1170. DOI: 10.1056/NEJM197512042932303.

5. Smith, D. C., R. Prentice, and D. J. Thomson, "Herrmann W.L. Association of exogenous estrogen and endogenous carcinoma." *N. Engl. J. Med.* 293 (1975): 1164–1167. DOI: 10.1056/NEJM197512042932302.

6. Woodruff, J. D., and J. H. Pickar. "Incidence of endometrial hyperplasia in postmenopausal women taking conjugated estrogens (Premarin) with medroxyprogesterone acetate or conjugated estrogens alone.

"The Menopause Study Group." *Am. J. Obstet. Gynecol.* 170 (1994): 1213–1223. DOI: 10.1016/S0002-9378(13)90437-3.

7.   Lobo, R. A. "Hormone-replacement therapy: Current thinking." *Nat. Rev. Endocrinol.* 13 (2017): 220–231. DOI: 10.1038/nrendo.2016.164.

8.   North American Menopause Society. "The 2012 hormone therapy position statement of the North American Menopause Society." *Menopause.* 19 (2012): 257–271. DOI: 10.1097/gme.0b013e31824b970a.

9.   Grodstein, F., et al. "Postmenopausal hormone therapy and mortality." *N. Engl. J. Med.* 336 (1997): 1769–1775. DOI: 10.1056/NEJM199706193362501.

10. Yaffe, K., et al. "Estrogen therapy in postmenopausal women: Effects on cognitive function and dementia." *JAMA* 279 (1998): 688–695. DOI: 10.1001/jama.279.9.688.

11. Stampfer, M. J., and G. A. Colditz. "Estrogen replacement therapy and coronary heart disease: A quantitative assessment of the epidemiologic evidence." *Prev. Med.* 20 (1991): 47–63. DOI: 10.1016/0091-7435(91)90006-P.

12. Grady, D., et al. "Hormone therapy to prevent disease and prolong life in postmenopausal women." *Ann. Intern. Med.* 117 (1992): 1016–1037. DOI: 10.7326/0003-4819-117-12-1016.

13. Lobo, R. A., et al. "Back to the future: Hormone replacement therapy as part of a prevention strategy for women at the onset of menopause." *Atherosclerosis.* 254 (2016): 296–304. DOI: 10.1016/j.atherosclerosis.2016.10.005.

14. American Medical Association Guidelines for counseling postmenopausal women about preventive hormone therapy." American College of Physicians. *Ann. Intern. Med.* 117 (1992): 1038–1041. DOI: 10.7326/0003-4819-117-12-1038.

15. Lobo, R. A., and M. Whitehead. "Too much of a good thing? Use of progestogens in the menopause: An international consensus statement." *Fertil. Steril.* 51 (1989): 229–231. DOI: 10.1016/S0015-0282(16)60481-8.

16. Shapiro, S., et al. "Does hormone replacement therapy cause breast cancer? An application of causal principles to three studies. Part 4: The Million Women Study." *Journal of Family Planning and Reproductive Health Care* 38(2) (Apr 2012): 102–109. DOI: 10.1136/jfprhc-2011-100229.

17. Manson, J. E., et al. "Menopausal hormone therapy and health out-
     comes during the intervention and extended poststopping phases of
     the Women's Health Initiative randomized trials." *JAMA* 310 (2013):
     1353–1368. DOI: 10.1001/jama.2013.278040.

18. Hsia, J., et al. "Women's Health Initiative Investigators. Conjugated
     equine estrogens and coronary heart disease: The Women's Health
     Initiative." *Arch. Intern. Med.* 166 (2006): 357–365. DOI: 10.1001/
     archinte.166.3.357.

19. Salpeter, S. R., et al. "Brief report: Coronary heart disease events
     associated with hormone therapy in younger and older women. A
     meta-analysis." *J. Gen. Intern. Med.* 21 (2006): 363–366. DOI: 10.1111/j.1
     525-1497.2006.00389.x.

20. Salpeter, S. R., et al. "Mortality associated with hormone replacement
     therapy in younger and older women: A meta-analysis." *J. Gen. Intern.
     Med.* 19 (2004): 791–804. DOI: 10.1111/j.1525-1497.2004.30281.x.

21. Boardman, H. M., et al. "Hormone therapy for preventing cardiovascu-
     lar disease in postmenopausal women." *Cochrane Database Syst. Rev.*
     (2015). DOI: 10.1002/14651858.CD002229.pub4.

22. Rossouw, J. E., et al. "Postmenopausal hormone therapy and car-
     diovascular disease by age and years since menopause." *JAMA* 297
     (2007): 1465–1477. DOI: 10.1001/jama.297.13.1465.

23. Schierbeck, L. L., et al. "Effect of hormone replacement therapy on car-
     diovascular events in recently postmenopausal women: Randomized
     trial." *BMJ* 345 (2012): e6409. DOI: 10.1136/bmj.e6409.

Chapter 2: What Are Hormones, and Why Do We Need Them?

24. Gaignard, P., et al. "The Role of Sex Hormones on Brain Mitochondrial
     Function, with Special Reference to Aging and Neurodegenerative
     Diseases." *Front. Aging Neurosci.* 9 (Dec 7, 2017): 406. DOI: 10.3389/
     fnagi.2017.00406.

Chapter 5: Progesterone

25. Zerr-Fouineau, M., et al. "Progestins overcome inhibition of platelet
     aggregation by endothelial cells by down-regulating endothelial NO
     synthase via glucocorticoid receptors." *Faseb J.* 21 (2007): 265–273.

26. Ghanderhari, S., et al. "Progesterone in Addition to Standard of Care vs Standard of Care Alone in the Treatment of Men Hospitalized with Moderate to Severe COVID-19: A Randomized, Controlled Pilot Trial." *Chest.* 160(1) (Jul 2021): 74–84.

Chapter 6: Estradiol and Progesterone Effects on the Brain

27. Cornil, C. A., G. F. Ball, and J. Balhazart. "Functional significance of the rapid regulation of brain estrogen action: where do estrogens come from?" *Brain Res.* 1126(1) (Dec 18 2006): 2–26. DOI: 10.1016/j.brainres.2006.07.098.

28. Holloway, C. C., and D. F. Clayton. "Estrogen synthesis in the mail brain triggers development of the avian song control pathway in vitro." *Nat Neurosci.* 4(2) (Feb 2001): 170–5.

29. Schlinger, B. A., and A. P. Arnold. "Circulating estrogens in a male songbird originate in the brain." *Proc Natl Acad Sci USA* 89(16) (Aug 15, 1992): 7650–3.

30. Garcia-Segura, L. M., et al. "Estradiol, insulin-like growth factor-I and brain aging." *Psychoneuroendocrinology.* 32 Suppl 1 (Aug 2007): S57–61.

31. van Amelsvoort, T., et al. "Prolactin response to d-fenfluramine in postmenopausal women on and off ERT: comparison with young women." *Psychoneuroendocrinology* 26 (2001): 493–502.

32. Shaywitz, S. E., et al. "Effect of estrogen on brain activation patterns in postmenopausal women during working memory tasks." *JAMA* 281(13) (Apr 7, 1999): 1197–202.

33. Xu, H., et al. "Estrogen reduces neuronal generation of Alzheimer beta-amyloid peptides." *Nat Med.* 4 (1998): 447–51.

34. Cutter, W. J., R. Norbury, and D. G. M. Murphy. "Oestrogen, brain function, and neuropsychiatric disorders." *Journal of Neurology, Neurosurgery & Psychiatry* 74 (2003): 837–840.

35. Asthan, S., et al. "High doses of estradiol improves cognition for women with AD: results of a randomized study." *Neurology* 57 (2001): 605–12.

36. Matyi, J. M., et al. "Lifetime exposure and cognition in later life: The Cache County Study." *Menopause.* 26(12) (Dec 2019): 1366–1374.

37. Phillips, S. M., and B. B. Sherwin. "Effects of estrogen on memory function in surgically menopausal women." *Psychoneuroendocrinology* 17 (1992): 485–95.

38. Sherwin, B. B. "Estrogen and/or androgen replacement therapy and cognitive functioning in surgically menopausal women." *Psychoneuroendocrinology* 13 (1988): 345–57.

39. Robertson, D. M., et al. "Effects of estrogen replacement therapy on human brain aging: And in vivo 1H MRS study." *Neurology* 57 (2001): 2114–17.

40. Amandusson, A., and A. Blomqvist. "Estrogenic influences in pain processing." *Frontiers in Neuroendocrinology* (34) (2013): 4329–349.

41. Smith, Y. R., et al. "Pronociceptive and antinociceptive effect of estradiol through endogenous opioid neurotransmission in women." *J Neurosci.* 26(21) (May 24, 2006): 5777–85.

42. Singh, M., et al. "Estrogen-induced activation of mitogen-activated protein kinase and cerebral cortical explants: convergence of estrogen and neurotrophin signaling pathways." *J Neurosci.* 19(4) (Feb 15, 1999): 1179–88.

43. Carrer, H. F., M. J. Cambiasso, and S. Gorosito. "Effects of estrogen on neuronal growth and differentiation." *J Steroid Biochem Mol Biol.* 93(2-5) (Feb 2005): 319–23.

44. Maki, P. M., and Resnick, S. M. "Longitudinal effects of estrogen replacement therapy on PET cerebral flow and cognition." *Neurobiol Aging.* 21(2) (Mar–Apr 2000): 373–83.

45. Behl, Christian. "Oestrogen as a neuroprotective hormone." *Nat Rev Neurosci.* 3(6) (Jun 2002): 433–42. DOI: 10.1038/nrn846.

46. Lord, C., et al. "Hippocampal volumes are larger in postmenopausal women using estrogen therapy compared to past users, never users and men: a possible window of opportunity effect." *Neurobiol. Aging* 29(1) (Jan 2008): 95–101.

47. Soares, C. N., et al. "Efficacy of estradiol for the treatment of depressive disorders in perimenopausal women: A double-blind, randomized, placebo controlled trial." *Arch Gen Psychiatry.* 58(6) (Jun 2001): 529–34.

48. Gordon, Jennifer L., et al. "Efficacy of Transdermal Estradiol and Micronized Progesterone in the Prevention of Depressive Symptoms in the Menopause Transition: A Randomized Clinical Trial." *JAMA Psychiatry* 75(2) (Feb 1, 2018): 149–157.

49. Baulieu, E., and M. Schumacher. "Progesterone as a neuroactive neurosteroid, with special reference to the effect of progesterone on myelination." *Steroids* 65(10–11) (Oct–Nov 2000): 605–612.

50. Berent-Spillson, A., et al. "Distinct cognitive effects of estrogen and progesterone in menopausal women." *Psychoneuroendocrinology* 59 (Sep 2015): 25–36.

51. Cohen, L.S., et al. "Risk for new onset of depression during the menopausal transition: the Harvard study of moods and cycles." *Arch. Gen. Psychiatry* 63 (2006a): 385–390. DOI: 10.1001/archpsyc.63.4.385.

52. Freeman, E. W., et al. "Associations of hormones and menopausal status with depressed mood in women with no history of depression." *Arch. Gen. Psychiatry* 63 (2006): 375–382. DOI: 10.1001/archpsyc.63.4.375.

53. Stein, D. W., D. W. Wright, and A. L. Kellermann. "Does progesterone have neuroprotective properties?" *Ann Emerg Med.* 51 (2008): 164–172.

54. Baulieu, E. E., and P. Robel. "Neurosteroids: a new brain function?" *J Steroid Biochem Mol Biol.* 37 (1990): 395–403.

55. Stein, D. G., and D. W. Wright. "Progesterone in the clinical treatment of acute traumatic brain injury." *Expert Opin Investig Drugs* 19 (2010): 847–857.

56. Espinoza, T. R., and D. W. Wright. "The role of progesterone and traumatic brain injury." *J Head Trauma Rehabil.* 26(6) (Nov–Dec 2011): 497–499.

57. Wright, D. W., et al. "ProTECT: a randomized clinical trial of progesterone for acute traumatic brain injury." *Ann Emerg Med.* 49 (2007): 391–402.

58. Xiao, G., et al. "Improved outcomes from the administration of progesterone for patients with acute severe traumatic brain injury: a randomized controlled trial." *Crit Care* 12 (2008): R61.

59. Baulieu, E., and M. Schumacher. "Progesterone as a neuroactive neurosteroid, with special reference to the effect of progesterone on myelination." *Steroids* 65 (2000): 605–612.

Chapter 7: Osteoporosis and Osteoarthritis

60. Alford, A. I., K. M. Kozloff, and K. D. Hankenson. "Extracellular matrix networks in bone remodeling." *Int. J. Biochem. Cell Biol.* 65 (2015): 20–31.

61. Oldknow, K. J., V. E. Macrae, and C. Farquharson. "Endocrine role of bone: Recent and emerging perspectives beyond osteocalcin." *J. Endocrinol.* 225 (2015): R1–R19.

62. Albright, F. "Post-menopausal osteoporosis." *Trans Assoc Am Physicians* 55 (1940): 298–305.

63. Bouillon, R., et al. "Estrogens Are Essential for Male Pubertal Periosteal Bone Expansion." *J. Clin. Endocrinol. Metab.* 89 (2004): 6025–6029.

64. Manolagas, S. C. "From Estrogen-Centric to Aging and Oxidative Stress: A Revised Perspective of the Pathogenesis of Osteoporosis." *Endocr. Rev.* 31 (2010): 266–300.

65. J.-P. Bonjour and T. Chevalley. "Pubertal Timing, Bone Acquisition, and Risk of Fracture Throughout Life." *Endocr. Rev.* 35 (2014): 820–847.

66. Johnell, O., et al. "Risk factors for hip fracture in European women: The MEDOS study." *J. Bone Miner. Res.* 10 (2009): 1802–1815.

67. Chevalley, T., et al. "Deleterious Effect of Late Menarche on Distal Tibia Microstructure in Healthy 20-Year-Old and Premenopausal Middle-Aged Women." *J. Bone Miner. Res.* 24 (2009): 144–152. DOI: 10.1359/jbmr.080815.

68. Vandenput, L., et al. "Pubertal timing and adult fracture risk in men: A population-based cohort study." *PLoS Med.* 16 (2019): e1002986.

69. Yeh, M.-C., et al. "Increased Risk of Sudden Sensorineural Hearing Loss in Patients with Osteoporosis: A Population-based, Propensity Score-matched, Longitudinal Follow-Up Study." *The Journal of Clinical Endocrinology & Metabolism,* 100(6) (Jun 2015): 2413–2419.

70. Oursler, M. J., et al. "Avian osteoclasts as estrogen target cells." *Proc Natl Acad Sci USA* 88 (1991): 6613–6617.

71. Nakamura, T., et al. "Estrogen prevents bone loss via estrogen receptor alpha and induction of fas ligand in osteoclasts." *Cell* 130 (2007): 811–823.

72. Martin-Millan, M., et al. "The estrogen receptor-alpha in osteoclasts mediates the protective effects of estrogens on cancellous but not cortical bone." *Mol Endocrinol.* 24 (2010): 323–334.

73. Iyer, S., et al. "ERalpha-deletion from osteoblast progenitors abolishes the protective effect of estrogens on cortical bone mass in both female and male mice." *J Bone Miner Res.* 26 (Suppl 1) (2011).

74. Bonewald, L. F. "The amazing osteocyte." *J Bone Miner Res.* 26 (2011): 229–238.

75. Kohrt, W. M., D. B. Snead, and E. Slatopolsky. "Additive effects of weight-bearing exercise and estrogen on bone mineral density in older women." *J Bone Miner Res.* 10(9) (Sep 1995): 1303–11.

76. Vico, L., et al. "Effects of long-term microgravity exposure on cancellous and cortical weight-bearing bones of cosmonauts." *Lancet* 355 (2000): 1607–1611.

77. Charatcharoenwitthaya, N., et al. "Effect of blockade of TNF-a and interleukin-1 action on bone resorption in early postmenopausal women." *J Bone Miner Res.* 22 (2007): 724–729.

78. Rogers, A., and R. Eastell. "Effects of estrogen therapy of postmenopausal women on cytokines measured in peripheral blood." *J Bone Miner Res.* 13(10) (Oct 1998): 1577–86.

79. Lindsey, R., et al. "Bone response to termination of oestrogen treatment." *Lancer* 1(8078) (June 24, 1978): 1325–7.

80. Sniekers, Y. H., et al. "Oestrogen is important for maintenance of cartilage and subchondral bone in a murine model of knee osteoarthritis." *Arthritis Res Ther.* 12 (2010): R182.

81. Li, G., et al. "Subchondral bone in osteoarthritis: insight into the risk factors and microstructural changes." *Arthritis Res Ther.* 15 (2013): 223.

Chapter 8: Skeletal Muscle, Tendons, and Ligaments

82. Enns, D. L., and P. M. Tidus. "The influence of estrogen on skeletal muscle: sex matters." *Sports Med.* 40(1) (Jan 1, 2010): 41–58.

83. Kitajima, Y., and Y. Ono. "Estrogens maintain skeletal muscle and satellite cell functions." *J. Endocrinol.* 229 (2016): 267–75.

84. Enns, D. L., and P. M. Tidus. "The influence of estrogen on skeletal muscle: sex matters." *Sports Med.* 40(1) (Jan 1, 2010): 41–58.

85. Smith, G. I., et al. "Testosterone and progesterone, but not estradiol, stimulate muscle protein synthesis in postmenopausal women." *J. Clin. Endocrinol. Metab.* 99 (2014): 256–265.

86. Taaffe, D. R., et al. "Estrogen replacement, muscle composition, and physical function: the health ABC study." *Med. Sci. Sports Exerc.* 37 (2005): 1741–1747.

87. Lee, C. Y., et al. "The combined regulation of estrogen and cyclic tension on fibroblast biosynthesis derived from anterior cruciate ligament." *Matrix Biol.* 23 (2004a): 323–329.

88. Dieli-Conwright, C. M., et al. "Influence of hormone replacement therapy on eccentric exercise induced myogenic gene expression in postmenopausal women." *J. Appl. Physiol.* 107 (2009): 1381–1388.

89. Pöllänen, E., et al. "Power training and postmenopausal hormone therapy affect transcriptional control of specific co-regulated gene clusters in skeletal muscle." *Age* 32 (2010): 347–363.

90. Ronkainen, P. H., et al. "Postmenopausal hormone replacement therapy modifies skeletal muscle composition and function: a study with monozygotic twin pairs." *J. Appl. Physiol.* 107 (2009): 25–33.

91. Sipilä, S., et al. "Effects of hormone replacement therapy and high-impact physical exercise on skeletal muscle in post-menopausal women: a randomized placebo-controlled study." *Clin. Sci.* 101 (2001): 147–157.

92. Hansen, M., et al. "Effect of administration of oral contraceptives on the synthesis and breakdown of myofibrillar proteins in young women." *Scand J Med Sci Sports* 21(1) (Feb 2011): 62–7.

93. Valencia, A. P., et al. "The presence of the ovary prevents hepatic mitochondrial oxidative stress in young and aged female mice through glutathione peroxidase 1." *Exp. Gerontol.* 73 (Jan 2016): 14–22.

94. Baltgalvis, K. A., et al. "Estrogen regulates estrogen receptors and antioxidant gene expression in mouse skeletal muscle." *PLoS ONE* 5(4) (Apr 2010): e10164. DOI: 10.1371/journal.pone.0010164.

95. Torres, M. J., et al. "17β-estradiol directly lowers mitochondrial membrane microviscosity and improves bioenergetic function in skeletal muscle." *Cell Metab.* 27 (2018): 167–179.

96. Spangenburg, E. E., et al. "Regulation of physiological and metabolic function of muscle by female sex steroids." *Med. Sci. Sports Exerc.* 44 (2012): 1653–1662.

97. Camporez, J. P., et al. "Cellular mechanism by which estradiol protects female ovariectomized mice from high-fat diet-induced hepatic and muscle insulin resistance." *Endocrinology* 154 (2013): 1021–1028.

98. Westh, E., et al. "Effect of habitual exercise on the structural and mechanical properties of human tendon, *in vivo*, in men and women." *Scand. J. Med. Sci. Sports* 18 (2008): 23–30.

99. Hansen, M., et al. "Effect of estrogen on tendon collagen synthesis, tendon structural characteristics, and biomechanical properties in postmenopausal women." *J. Appl. Physiol.* 106 (2009b): 1385–1393.

100. Lee, C. Y., et al. "Tensile forces attenuate estrogen-stimulated collagen synthesis in the ACL." *Biochem. Biophys. Res. Commun.* 317 (2004b): 1221–1225.

101. Miller, B. F., et al. "No effect of menstrual cycle on myofibrillar and connective tissue protein synthesis in contracting skeletal muscle." *Am. J. Physiol. Endocrinol. Metabol.* 290 (2006): E163–E168.

102. Magnusson, S. P., et al. "The adaptability of tendon to loading differs in men and women." *Int. J. Exp. Pathol.* 88 (2007): 237–240.

103. Hansen, M., et al. "Effect of estrogen on tendon collagen synthesis, tendon structural characteristics, and biomechanical properties in postmenopausal women." *J. Appl. Physiol.* 106 (2009b): 1385–1393.

104. West, D. W., et al. "The exercise-induced biochemical milieu enhances collagen content and tensile strength of engineered ligaments." *J. Physiol.* 593 (2015): 4665–4675.

105. Hansen, M., et al. "Local administration of insulin-like growth factor-1 (IGF-1) stimulates tendon collagen synthesis in humans." *Scand. J. Med. Sci. Sports* 23 (2013): 614–619.

106. Hansen, M. "Female hormones: do they influence muscle and tendon protein metabolism?" *Proc. Nutr. Soc.* 77 (2018): 32–41.

107. Dieli-Conwright, C. M., et al. "Influence of hormone replacement therapy on eccentric exercise induced myogenic gene expression in postmenopausal women." *J Applied Physiol (1985)* 107(5) (Nov 2009): 1381–8.

Chapter 9: Estradiol and Cardiovascular Health

108. Bagot, C. N., et al. "The effect of estrone on thrombin generation may explain the different thrombotic risk between oral and transdermal hormone replacement therapy." *Journal of Thrombosis and Haemostasis* 8 (2010): 1736–1744.

109. Knowlton, A. A., and A. R. Lee. "Estrogen and the cardiovascular system." *Pharmacol Ther* 135(1) (Jul 2012): 54–70.

110. Donato, A. J., et al. "Aging is associated with greater nuclear NFκB, reduced IκBα, and increased expression of proinflammatory cytokines in vascular endothelial cells of healthy humans." *Aging Cell* 7 (2008): 805–812.

111. Booth, E. A., and B. R. Lucchesi. "Estrogen-Mediated Protection in Myocardial Ischemia-Reperfusion Injury." *Cardiovascular Toxicology* 8 (2008): 101–113.

112. Siow, R. C. M., et al. "Cardiovascular targets for estrogens and phytoestrogens: Transcriptional regulation of nitric oxide synthase and antioxidant defense genes." *Free Radical Biology and Medicine* 42 (2007): 909–925.

113. Booth, E. A., et al. "17{beta}-Estradiol as a Receptor-Mediated Cardioprotective Agent." *Journal of Pharmacology and Experimental Therapeutics* 307 (2003): 395–401.

114. Bader, A., et al. "Oestrogènes naturels et système cardio-vasculaire [Natural estrogens and the cardiovascular system]." *J Gynecol Obstet Biol Reprod (Paris)* 25(3) (1996): 233–7. French. PMID: 8767217.

115. Schulz, E., et al. "Estradiol-mediated endothelial nitric oxide synthase association with heat shock protein 90 requires adenosine monophosphate-dependent protein kinase." *Circulation* 111(25) (Jun 2005): 3473–80. DOI: 10.1161/CIRCULATIONAHA.105.546812.

116. Chan, G., and R. Fiscus. "Exaggerated production of nitric oxide (NO) and increases in inducible NO-synthase mRNA levels induced by the

pro-inflammatory cytokine interleukin-1β in vascular smooth muscle cells of elderly rats." *Experimental Gerontology* 39 (2004): 387–394.

117. Sowers, J. R. "Diabetes Melitus and Cardiovascular Disease in Women." *Archives of Internal Medicine* 158 (1998): 617–621.

118. Haynes, M. P., et al. "Membrane estrogen receptor engagement activates endothelial nitric oxide synthase via the PI3-Kinase-Akt pathway in human endothelial cells." *Circulation Research* 87 (2000): 677–682

119. Hisamoto, K., et al. "Estrogen Induces the Akt-dependent Activation of Endothelial Nitric-oxide Synthase in Vascular Endothelial Cells." *Journal of Biological Chemistry* 276 (2001): 3459–3467.

120. Novensa, L., et al. "Equine Estrogens Impair Nitric Oxide Production and Endothelial Nitric Oxide Synthase Transcription in Human Endothelial Cells Compared with the Natural 17β-estradiol." *Hypertension* 56 (2010): 405–411.

121. Wingrove, C. S., et al. "Effects of equine oestrogens on markers of vasoactive function in human coronary artery endothelial cells." *Molecular and Cellular Endocrinology* 150 (1999): 33–37.

122. Ling, S., et al. "High glucose abolishes the antiproliferative effect of 17beta-estradiol in human vascular smooth muscle cells." *Am J Physiol Endocrinol Metab.* 282(4) (Apr 2002): E746–51. DOI: 10.1152/ajpendo.00111.2001.

123. Pare, G., et al. "Estrogen Receptor-α Mediates the Protective Effects of Estrogen Against Vascular Injury." *Circ Res* 90 (2002): 1087–1092.

124. Dubey, R. K., et al. "Clinically Used Estrogens Differentially Inhibit Human Aortic Smooth Muscle Cell Growth and Mitogen-Activated Protein Kinase Activity." *Arteriosclerosis, Thrombosis, and Vascular Biology* 20 (2000): 964–972.

125. Gupte, A. A., H. J. Pownall, and D. J. Hamilton. "Estrogen: an emerging regulator of insulin action and mitochondrial function." *J Diabetes Res* 2015 (Mar 2015): 916585. DOI: 10.1155/2015/916585.

126. Carr, M. C. "The emergence of the metabolic syndrome with menopause." *J Clin Endocrinol Metab.* 88 (2003): 2404–11.

127. Xing, D., et al. "Estrogen and Mechanisms of Vascular Protection." *Arteriosclerosis, Thrombosis, and Vascular Biology* 29 (2009): 289–295.

128. Parini, P., B. Angelin, and M. Rudlin. "Importance of Estrogen Receptors in Hepatic LDL Receptor Regulation." *Arteriosclerosis, Thrombosis, and Vascular Biology* 17 (1997): 1800–1805.

129. Simoncini, T., R. De Caterina, and A. R. Genazzani. "Selective Estrogen Receptor Modulators: Different Actions on Vascular Cell Adhesion Molecule-1 (VCAM-1) Expression in Human Endothelial Cells." *Journal of Clinical Endocrinology Metabolism* 84 (1999): 815.

130. Rodriguez, E., et al. "17[beta]-estradiol inhibits the adhesion of leukocytes in TNF-[alpha] stimulated human endothelial cells by blocking IL-8 and MCP-1 secretion, but not its transcription." *Life Sciences* 71 (2002): 2181–2193.

131. Karas, R. H., et al. "Effects of Estrogen on the Vascular Injury Response in Estrogen Receptor α,β (Double) Knockout Mice." *Circ Res* 89 (2001): 534–539.

132. Keung, W., et al. "Non-genomic activation of adenylyl cyclase and protein kinase G by 17β-estradiol in vascular smooth muscle of the rat superior mesenteric artery." *Pharmacological Research* 64 (2011): 509–516.

133. Kim, J. K., et al. "Estrogen Prevents Cardiomyocyte Apoptosis through Inhibition of Reactive Oxygen Species and Differential Regulation of p38 Kinase Isoforms." *Journal of Biological Chemistry* 281 (2006a): 6760–6767.

134. Nakamura, Y., T. Suzuki, and H. Sasano. "Estrogen actions and in situ synthesis in human vascular smooth muscle cells and their correlation with atherosclerosis." *J Steroid Biochem Mol Biol* 93(2-5) (Feb 2005): 263–8.

135. Nakamura, Y., et al. "Estrogen receptors in atherosclerotic human aorta: inhibition of human vascular smooth muscle cell proliferation by estrogens." *Molecular and Cellular Endocrinology* 219 (2004): 17–26.

136. Kim, K. H., and J. R. Bender. "Membrane-initiated actions of estrogen on the endothelium." *Molecular and Cellular Endocrinology* 308 (2009): 3–8.

137. Luo, T., and J. K. Kim. "The Role of Estrogen and Estrogen Receptors on Cardiomyocytes: An Overview." *Can J Cardiol.* 32(8) (Aug 2016): 1017–25.

138. Devanathan, S., et al. "An animal model with a cardiomyocyte-specific deletion of estrogen receptor alpha: Functional, metabolic, and differential network analysis." *PloS One* 9 (2014): e101900.

139. Chen, Y., et al. "17beta-estradiol prevents cardiac diastolic dysfunction by stimulating mitochondrial function: A preclinical study in a mouse model of a human hypertrophic cardiomyopathy mutation." *J Steroid Biochem Mol Biol.* 147 (2015): 92–102.

140. Pelzer, T., et al. "17beta-estradiol prevents programmed cell death in cardiac myocytes." *Biochem Biophys Res Commun* 268 (2000): 192–200.

141. Pelzer, T., et al. "Estrogen effects in the myocardium: Inhibition of NF-kappab DNA binding by estrogen receptor-alpha and -beta." *Biochem Biophys Res Commun* 286 (2001): 1153–7.

142. Patten, R. D., et al. "17beta-estradiol reduces cardiomyocyte apoptosis in vivo and in vitro via activation of phospho-inositide-3 kinase/Akt signaling." *Circ Res* 95 (2004): 692–9.

143. Satoh, M., et al. "Inhibition of apoptosis-regulated signaling kinase-1 and prevention of congestive heart failure by estrogen." *Circulation* 115 (2007): 3197–204.

144. Cong, B., et al. "Estrogens protect myocardium against ischemia/reperfusion insult by up-regulation of CRH receptor type 2 in female rats." *Int J Cardiol* 168 (2013): 4755–60.

145. Liu, H., et al. "Mitochondrial p38beta and manganese superoxide dismutase interaction mediated by estrogen in cardiomyocytes." *PloS One* 9 (2014): e85272.

146. Liu, H., A. Pedram, and J. K. Kim. "Oestrogen prevents cardiomyocyte apoptosis by suppressing p38alpha-mediated activation of p53 and by down-regulating p53 inhibition on p38beta." *Cardiovasc Res* 89 (2011): 119–28.

147. Kim, J. K., et al. "Estrogen prevents cardiomyocyte apoptosis through inhibition of reactive oxygen species and differential regulation of p38 kinase isoforms." *J Biol Chem.* 281 (2006): 6760–7.

148. Liou, C. M., et al. "Effects of 17beta-estradiol on cardiac apoptosis in ovariectomized rats." *Cell Biochem Funct* 28 (2010): 521–8.

149. Wang, L., et al. "Estradiol treatment promotes cardiac stem cell (CSC)-derived growth factors, thus improving CSC-mediated cardioprotection after acute ischemia/reperfusion." *Surgery* 156 (2014): 243–52.

150. Han, H. J., J. S. Heo, and Y. J. Lee. "Estradiol-17beta stimulates proliferation of mouse embryonic stem cells: Involvement of MAPKs and CDKs as well as protooncogenes." *Am J Physiol Cell Physiol* 290 (2006): C1067–75.

151. Hamada, H., et al. "Estrogen receptors alpha and beta mediate contribution of bone marrow-derived endothelial progenitor cells to functional recovery after myocardial infarction." *Circulation* 114 (2006): 2261–70.

Chapter 10: Estradiol and Progesterone Effects on the Immune System

152. K. Yuki, et al. "Review article COVID-19 pathophysiology: a review." *Clin Immunol* 215 (2020): 1–8.

153. Zhou, M., X. Zhang, and J. Qu. "Coronavirus disease 2019 (COVID-19): a clinical update." *Front Med* 14 (2020): 126–135.

154. Straub, R. H. "The complex role of estrogens in inflammation." *Endocr Rev.* 28(5) (2007): 521–574.

155. Cutolo, M., V. Smith, and S. Paolino. "Editorial: understanding immune effects of oestrogens to explain the reduced morbidity and mortality in female versus male COVID-19 patients. Comparisons with autoimmunity and vaccination." *Clin Exp Rheumatol* 38 (2020): 383–386.

156. Furman, D., et al. "Systems analysis of sex differences reveals an immunosuppressive role for testosterone in the response to influenza vaccination." *Proc Natl Acad Sci U S A* 111 (2014): 869–874.

157. Kamada, M., et al. "B cell subsets in postmenopausal women and the effect of hormone replacement therapy." *Maturitas* 37 (2001): 173–179.

158. Hoffmann, M., et al. "SARS-CoV-2 cell entry depends on ACE2 and TMPRSS2 and is blocked by a clinically proven protease inhibitor." *Cell* 181 (2020): 271–280.

159. Kovats, S. "Estrogen receptors regulate innate immune cells and signaling pathways." *Cell Immunol* 294 (2015): 63–69.

160. Freer, G., and D. Matteucci. "Influence of dendritic cells on viral pathogenicity." *PLOS Pathog* 5(7) (Jul 2009): e1000384.

161. Hall, O. J., et al. "Progesterone-based therapy protects against influenza by promoting lung repair and recovery in females." *PloS Pathog.* 12(9) (2016): e1005840.

162. Hall, O. J., et al. "Progesterone-based therapy protects against influenza by promoting lung repair and recovery in females." *PLoS Pathog* 12 (2016): 1–22.

163. Arruvito, L., et al. "NK cells expressing a progesterone receptor are susceptible to progesterone-induced apoptosis." *J Immunol* 180 (2008): 5746–5753.

164. Gordon, D. E., et al. "A SARS-CoV-2 protein interaction map reveals targets for drug repurposing." *Nature* 583 (2020): 459–468.

165. Chousterman, B. G., F. K. Swirski, and G. F. Weber. "Cytokine storm and sepsis disease pathogenesis." *Semin Immunopathol* 39(5) (2017): 517–528.

166. Ye Q., B. Wang, and J. Mao. "The pathogenesis and treatment of the 'Cytokine Storm' in COVID-19." *J Infect.* 80(6) (2020): 607–613.

167. Chen, G., et al. "Clinical and immunological features of severe and moderate coronavirus disease 2019." *J Clin Invest.* 130(5) (2020): 2620–2629.

168. Mehta, P., et al. "HLH Across Speciality Collaboration, UK. COVID-19: consider cytokine storm syndromes and immunosuppression." *Lancet* 395(10229) (2020): 1033–1034.

169. Ramírez-de-Arellano, A., et al. "The role of estradiol in the immune response against COVID-19." *Hormones* 20 (2021): 657–667.

170. Global Health 50/50. "The COVID-19 sex-disaggregated data tracker." Updated June 13, 2022. Available at: https://globalhealth5050.org/the-sex-gender-and-covid-19-project/the-data-tracker/. Accessed Sept. 9, 2022.

171. Marina, Scavini, and Lorenzo Piemonti. "Gender and Age Effects on the Rates of Infection and Deaths in Individuals with Confirmed SARS-CoV-2 Infection in Six European Countries." April 8, 2020. Available at: https://papers.ssrn.com/sol3/papers.cfm?abstract_id=3576790. Accessed Sept. 9, 2022.

172. Karlberg, J., D. S. Chong, and W. Y. Lai. "Do men have a higher case fatality rate of severe acute respiratory syndrome than women do?" *Am J Epidemiol* 159(3) (2004): 229–23.

173. Alghamdi, I. G., et al. "The pattern of middle east respiratory syndrome coronavirus in Saudi Arabia: a descriptive epidemiological analysis of data from the Saudi Ministry of Health." *Int J Gen Med.* 7 (2014): 417–423.

174. Zeng, F., et al. "A comparison study of SARS-CoV-2 IgG antibody between male and female COVID-19 patients: a possible reason underlying different outcome between sex." *J Med Virol* 92 (2020): 2050–2054.

175. Lu, R., et al. "Genomic characterization and epidemiology of 2019 novel coronavirus: implications for virus origins and receptor binding." *Lancet* 395 (2020) :565–574.

176. K. Yuki, et al. "Review article COVID-19 pathophysiology: a review." *Clin Immunol* 215 (2020): 1–8.

177. M. Zhou, X. Zhang, and J. Qu. "Coronavirus disease 2019 (COVID-19): a clinical update." *Front Med* 14 (2020): 126–135.

178. Lee, C.-H., et al. "Altered p38 mitogen-activated protein kinase expression in different leukocytes with increment of immunosuppressive mediators in patients with severe acute respiratory syndrome." *J Immunol* 172 (2004): 7841–7847.

179. Glinsky, G. V. "Tripartite combination of candidate pandemic mitigation agents: vitamin D, quercetin, and estradiol manifest properties of medicinal agents for targeted mitigation of the COVID-19 pandemic defined by genomics-guided tracing of SARS-CoV-2 targets in human." *Biomedicines* 8 (2020): 129.

180. Hoffmann, M., et al. "SARS-CoV-2 cell entry depends on ACE2 and TMPRSS2 and is blocked by a clinically proven protease inhibitor." *Cell* 181 (2020): 271–280.

181. Stelzig, K. E., et al. "Estrogen regulates the expression of SARS-CoV-2 receptor ACE2 in differentiated airway epithelial cells." *Am J Physiol Cell Mol Physiol* 318 (2020): L1280–L1281.

182. Cantenys-Molina, S., et al. "Lymphocyte subsets early predict mortality in a large series of hospitalized COVID-19 patients in Spain." *Clin Exp Immunol* 203(3) (Mar 2020): 424–432. DOI: 10.1111/cei.13547.

183. Di Stadio, A., et al. "Gender differences in COVID-19 infection. The estrogen effect on upper and lower airways. Can it help to figure out a treatment?" *Eur Rev Med Pharmacol Sci* 24(10) (May 2020): 5195–5196.

184. Chen, H., et al. "Clinical characteristics and intrauterine vertical transmission potential of COVID-19 infection in nine pregnant women: a retrospective review of medical records." *Lancet* 395 (2020): 809–815.

185. Dana, P., et al. "COVID-19 and pregnancy: a review of current knowledge." *Infez Med.* 28(suppl 1) (Jun 2020): 46–51.

186. Breithaupt-Faloppa, A. C., et al. "17β-Estradiol, a potential ally to alleviate SARS-CoV-2 infection." *Clinics (Sao Paulo)* 75 (2020): e1980. DOI: 10.6061/clinics/2020/e1980.

187. Grandi, G., F. Facchinetti, and J. Bitzer. "The gendered impact of coronavirus disease (COVID-19): do estrogens play a role?" *Eur J Contracept Reprod Health Care* 25 (2020): 233–234.

188. Shi, L., et al. "Role of estrogen in hepatocellular carcinoma: is inflammation the key?" *J Transl Med.* 12 (Apr 2014): 93. DOI: 10.1186/1479-5876-12-93.

189. Di Martino, V., et al. "Progression of liver fibrosis in women infected with hepatitis C: long-term benefit of estrogen exposure." *Hepatology* 40(6) (2004): 1426–1433.

Chapter 11: Testosterone in Men

190. Kloner, R. A., et al. "Testosterone and Cardiovascular Disease." *J Am Coll Cardiol.* 67(5) (Feb 9, 2016): 545–5.

191. Celec, P., D. Ostatnikova, and J. Hodosy. "On the effects of testosterone on brain behavioral functions." *Front Neurosci.* 9 (Feb 17, 2015): 12.

192. Carrier, N., et al. "The Anxiolytic and Antidepressant-like Effects of Testosterone and Estrogen in Gonadectomized Male Rats." *Biol Psychiatry* 78(4) (Aug 15, 2015): 259–69.

193. Gaignard, P., et al. "The Role of Sex Hormones on Brain Mitochondrial Function, with Special Reference to Aging and Neurodegenerative Diseases." *Front. Aging Neurosci.* 9 (Dec 7, 2017): 406.

194. Toma, M., et al. "Testosterone supplementation in heart failure: a meta-analysis." *Circ Heart Fail.* 5(3) (May 1, 2012): 315–2.

195. Jankowska, E. A., et al. "Anabolic deficiency in men with chronic heart failure: prevalence and detrimental impact on survival." *Circulation.* 114(17) (Oct 24, 2006): 1829–37.

196. Wehr, E., et al. "Low free testosterone is associated with heart failure mortality in older men referred for coronary angiography." *Eur J Heart Fail.* 13(5) (May 2011): 482–8.

197. Araujo, A. B., et al. "Clinical review: Endogenous testosterone and mortality in men: a systematic review and meta-analysis." *J Clin Endocrinol Metab.* 96(10) (Oct 2011): 3007–19.

198. Webb, C. M., et al. "Effects of testosterone on coronary vasomotor regulation in men with coronary heart disease." *Circulation* 100(16) (1999): 1690–6

199. Dos Santos, M. R., et al. "Effect of Exercise Training and Testosterone Replacement on Skeletal Muscle Wasting in Patients With Heart Failure With Testosterone Deficiency." *Mayo Clin Proc.* 91(5) (May 2016): 575–86.

200. Webb, C. M., et al. "Effect of acute testosterone on myocardial ischemia in men with coronary artery disease." *Am J Cardiol.* 83(3) (Feb 1, 1999): 437–9, A9.

201. Rosano, G. M., et al. "Acute anti-ischemic effect of testosterone in men with coronary artery disease." *Circulation* 99(13) (Apr 6, 1999): 1666–70.

202. English, K. M., et al. "Low-dose transdermal testosterone therapy improves angina threshold in men with chronic stable angina: A randomized, double-blind, placebo-controlled study." *Circulation* 102(16) (Oct 17, 2000): 1906–11.

203. Goodale, T., et al. "Testosterone and the Heart." *Methodist DeBakey Cardiovasc J.* 13(2) (Apr–Jun 2017): 68–72.

204. Kupelian, V., et al. "Inverse Association of Testosterone and the Metabolic Syndrome in Men is Consistent across Race and Ethnic Groups." *J Endocrinol Metab.* 93(9) (2008): 3403–3410.

205. Morgentaler, A., et al. "Testosterone therapy and cardiovascular risk: advances and controversies." *Mayo Clin Proc.* 90(2) (Feb 2015): 224–51.

206. Moradi, F. "Changes of Serum Adiponectin and Testosterone Concentrations Following Twelve Weeks of Resistance Training in Obese Young Men." *Asian J Sports Med.* 6(4) (Dec 6, 2015): e23808.

207. Dhindsa, S., et al. "Insulin Resistance and Inflammation in Hypogonadotropic Hypogonadism and Their Reduction After Testosterone Replacement in Men With Type 2 Diabetes." *Diabetes Care* 39(1) (Jan 2016): 82–91.

208. Kalinchenko, S. Y., et al. "Effects of testosterone supplementation on markers of the metabolic syndrome and inflammation in hypogonadal men with the metabolic syndrome: the double-blinded placebo-controlled Moscow study." *Clin Endocrinol (Oxf)*. 73(5) (Nov 2010): 602–12.

209. Heufelder, A. E., et al. "Fifty-two-week treatment with diet and exercise plus transdermal testosterone reverses the metabolic syndrome and improves glycemic control in men with newly diagnosed type 2 diabetes and subnormal plasma testosterone." *J Androl*. 30(6) (Nov–Dec 2009): 726–33.

210. Sinnesael M., et al. "Testosterone and the male skeleton: a dual mode of action." *Journal of Osteoporosis* (2011): 240328. DOI: 10.4061/2011/240328.

211. Herbst, K. and S. Bhasin. "Testosterone action on skeletal muscle." *Curr Opin Clin Nutr Metab Care* 7(3) (May 2004): 271–7.

212. Tehranipour, M. and A. Moghimi. "Neuroprotective effects of testosterone on regenerating spinal cord motor neurons in rats." *J Mot Behav*. 42(3) (May–Jun 2010): 151–5.

213. Bialek, M., et al. "Neuroprotective role of testosterone in the nervous system." *Pol J Pharmacol*. 56(5) (Sep–Oct 2004): 509–18.

214. Fernández-Balsells, M. M., et al. "Clinical review 1: Adverse effects of testosterone therapy in adult men: a systematic review and meta-analysis." *J Clin Endocrinol Metab*. 95(6) (June 2010): 2560–75.

215. Yeap, B. B., et al. "Lower Testosterone Levels Predict Incident Stroke and Transient Ischemic Attacks in Older Men." *J Clin Endocrinol Metab*. 94(7) (2008): 2353–2359.

216. Holmegard, H. N., et al. "Endogenous sex hormones and risk of venous thromboembolism in women and men." *J Thromb Haemost*. 12(3) (2014): 297–305.

217. Smith, A. M., et al. "Testosterone does not adversely affect fibrinogen or tissue plasminogen activator (tPA) and plasminogen activator

inhibitor-1 (PAI-1) levels in 46 men with chronic stable angina." *Eur J Endocrinol.* 152(2) (Feb 2005): 285–9.

Chapter 12: Prostate Cancer, BPH, and Testosterone

218. Wang, C., et al. "Investigation, treatment, and monitoring of late-onset hypogonadism in males: ISA, ISSAM, EAU, EAA, and ASA recommendations." *Eur Urol* 55(1) (Jan 2009): 121–30. DOI: 10.1016/j.eururo.2008.08.033.

219. Haider A., et al. "Incidence of prostate cancer in hypogonadal men receiving testosterone therapy: observation from 5-year median follow-up of 3 registries." *J Urol.* 193(1) (Jan 2015): 80–6.

220. Boyle, P., et al. "Endogenous and exogenous testosterone and the risk of prostate cancer and increased prostate-specific antigen (PSA) level: a meta-analysis." *BJU Int.* 118(5) (Nov 2016): 731–41.

221. Kaplan, A. L., and J. C. Hu. "Use of testosterone therapy in the United States and its effects on subsequent prostate cancer outcomes." *Urology* 82(2) (2013): 321–6.

222. Goren, M., and Y. Gat. "Varicocele is the root cause of BPH: destruction of the valves in spermatic veins produces elevated pressure which diverts undiluted testosterone directly from the testes to the prostate." *Andrologia* 50(5) (Jun 2008): e12992. DOI: 10.1111/and.12992.

Chapter 14: Breast Cancer

223. Lieberman, Allan, et al. "In Defense of Progesterone: A Review of the Literature." *Altern Ther Health Med.* 23(6) (Nov 2017): 24–32.

224. Campagnoli, Carlo, et al. "Progestins and progesterone in hormone replacement therapy and the risk of breast cancer." *J Steroid Biochem Mol Biol.* 96(2) (Jul 2005): 95–108.

225. Mauvais-Jarvis, P., F. Kuttenn, and A. Gompel. "Antiestrogenic action of progesterone in breast tissue." *Breast Cancer Res Treat.* 8(3) (1986): 179–88.

226. Vassilopoulou-Sellin, R., et al. "Estrogen Replacement Therapy After Localized Breast Cancer: Clinical Outcome of 319 Women Followed Prospectively." *J Clin Oncol.* 17(5) (1999): 1482–7.

227. Vassilopoulou-Sellin, R., et al. "Estrogen replacement therapy for menopausal woman with a history of breast carcinoma: Results of a 5-year, prospective study." *Cancer.* 2002 Nov 1;95(9): 1817–26.

228. Peters, G. N., et al. "Estrogen replacement therapy after breast cancer: A 12-year follow-up." *Ann Surg Onc.* 8(10) (Dec 2001): 828–32.

Chapter 15: Thyroid Gland

229. van Hoek , I., and S. Daminet. "Interactions between thyroid and kidney function in pathological conditions of these organ systems: a review." *Gen Comp E Endocrinol.* 160(3) (2009): 205–15.

230. Iglesias, P., and J. J. Diez. "Thyroid dysfunction and kidney disease." *Eur J Endocrinol.* 160(4) (2009): 503–15.

231. Portman, M. A. "Thyroid Hormone Regulation of Heart Metabolism." *Thyroid* 18(2) (2008): 217–25.

232. Danzi, S., and I. Klein. "Thyroid hormone-regulated cardiac gene expression and cardiovascular disease." *Thyroid* 12(6) (2022): 467–72.

233. Oetting, A., and P. M. Yen. "New insight into thyroid hormone action." *Best Pract Res Clin Endocrinol Metab.* 21(2) (2007): 193–208.

234. Malik, R., and H. Hodgson. "The relationship between the thyroid gland and the liver." *QJM* 95(9) (2002): 559–69.

235. Psarra, A. M., and C. E. Sekeris. "Steroid and thyroid hormone receptors in mitochondria." *IUBMB Life* 60(4) (2008): 210–23.

236. Scheller, K., P. Seibel, and C. E. Sekeris. "Glucocorticoid and thyroid hormone receptors in mitochondria of animal cell." *Int Rev Cytol.* 222 (2003): 1–61.

237. Psarra, A. M., S. Solakidi, and C. E. Sekeris. "The mitochondrion as a primary site of action of steroid and thyroid hormones: Presence and action of steroid and thyroid hormone receptors in mitochondria of animal cells." *Mol Cell Endocrinol.* 246(1-2) (2006): 21–33.

238. O'Brian, T., et al. "Hyperlipidemia in patients with primary and secondary hypothyroidism." *N Engl J Med.* 328 (1993): 1069–1075.

239. Goumidi, L., et al. "Study of thyroid hormone receptor alpha gene polymorphisms on Alzheimer's disease." *Neurobiol Aging* 32(4) (Apr 2011): 624–30.

240. Kelly, T., and D. Z. Lieberman. "The use of triiodothyronine as an agent in treatment resistant bipolar II disorders NOS." *Affect Disord.* 116(3) (Aug 2009): 222–6.

241. Nunez, J., et al. "Multigenic control of thyroid hormone functions in the nervous system." *Mol Cell Endocrinol.* 287 (1-2) (2008): 1–12.

242. Anderson, G. W. "Thyroid Hormone and Cerebellar development." *Cerebellum* 7(1) (2008): 60–74.

243. Ruggeri, R. M., et al. "Subacute thyroiditis in a patient infected with SARS-COV-2: an endocrine complication linked to the COVID-19 pandemic." *Hormones* 20 (2021): 219–221.

Chapter 16: Adrenal Glands

244. Susan P. Porterfield and Bruce A. White. *Endocrine Physiology.* 3rd ed. Mosby, Inc; 2007: 180.

245. David G. Gardner and Dolores Shoback. *Greenspan's Basic & Clinical Endocrinology.* 8th ed. McGraw-Hill Companies, Inc; 2007: 540.

Chapter 17: Growth Hormone

246. Rosenfeld, Ron G. "The future of research into growth hormone responsiveness." *Horm Res.* 71(Suppl 2) (2009): 71–4. DOI: 10.1159/000192440.

247. Woodhouse, Linda J., et al. "The influence of growth hormone status on physical impairments, functional limitations, and health-related quality of life in adults." *Endocr Rev.* 27(3) (2006): 287–317.

248. Rudman, D., et al. "Effects of human growth hormone in men over 60 years old." *N Eng J Med.* 323(1) (1990): 1–6. DOI: 10.1056/NEJM199007053230101.

249. Surya, Sowmya, et al. "The pattern of growth hormone delivery to peripheral tissues determines insulin-like growth factor-1 and lipolytic responses in obese subjects." *J Clin Endocrinol Metab.* 94(8) (2009): 2828–34. DOI: 10.1210/jc.2009-0638.

250. Kato, Keiko, et al. "Distinct role of growth hormone on epilepsy progression in a model of temporal lobe epilepsy." *J Neurochem.* 110(2) (2009): 509–19. DOI: 10.1111/j.1471-4159.2009.06132.x.

251. Chrisoulidou, A., et al. "How much, and by what mechanisms, does growth hormone replacement improve the quality of life in GH-deficient adults?" *Baillieres Clin Endocrinol Metab.* 12(2) (1998): 261–79. DOI: 10.1016/s0950-351x(98)80022-0.

252. Wallymahmed, M. E., et al. "Quality of life, body composition and muscle strength in adult growth hormone deficiency: the influence of growth hormone replacement therapy for up to 3 years." *Clin Endocrinol (Oxf).* 47(4) (1997): 439–46. DOI: 10.1046/j.1365-2265.1997.2 801076.x.

253. Muniyappa, Ranganath, et al. "Long-term testosterone supplementation augments overnight growth hormone secretion in healthy older men." *Am J Physiol Endocrinol Metab.* 293(3) (2007): E769–75. DOI: 10.1152/ajpendo.00709.2006.

254. Sattler, Fred R., et al. "Testosterone and growth hormone improve body composition and muscle performance in older men." *J Clin Endocrinol Metab.* 94(6) (1991–2001): 2008–2338. DOI: 10.1210/jc.2008-2338.

255. Vermeulen, A., S. Goemaere, and J. M. Kaufman. "Testosterone, body composition and aging." *J Endocrinol Invest.* 22(5Suppl) (1999): 110–6.

256. Vermeulen, Alex. "Aging, hormones, body composition, metabolic effects." *World J Urol.* 20(1) (2002): 23–7. DOI: 10.1007/s00345-002-0257-4.

257. Cuatrecasas, Guillem. "Fibromyalgic syndromes: could growth hormone therapy be beneficial?" *Pediatr Endocrinol Rev.* 6 Suppl 4 (Jun 2009): 529–33.

258. Sanders, Esmond J., Eve Parker, and Steve Harvey. "Endogenous growth hormone in human retinal ganglion cells correlates with cell survival." *Mol Vis.* 15 (2009): 920–6.

259. Morrhaye, Gabriel, et al. "Impact of growth hormone (GH) deficiency and GH replacement upon thymus function in adult patients." *PLos One* 4(5) (2009): e5668. DOI: 10.1371/journal.pone.0005668.

260. Leung, Kin-Chuen, et al. "Estrogen regulation of growth hormone action." *Endocr Rev.* 25 (2004): 693–721. DOI: 10.1210/er.2003-0035.

261. Veldhuis, Johannes D., and Cyril Y. Bowers. "Determinants of GH-releasing hormone and GH-releasing peptide synergy in men." *Am J Physiol Endocrinol Metab*. 296 (2009): E1085–1092. DOI: 10.1152/ajpendo.91001.2008.

262. Weltman, A., et al. "Relationship between age, percentage body fat, fitness, and 24-hour growth hormone release in healthy young adults: effects of gender." *J Clin Endocrinol Metab*. 78 (1994): 543–548.

263. Veldhuis, Johannes D., et al. "Relative effects of estrogen, age and visceral fat on pulsatile growth hormone secretion in healthy women." *Am J Physiol Endocrinol Metab*. 297(2) (2009): E367–74.

264. Veldhuis, Johannes D., et al. "Regulation of basal, pulsatile, and entropic (patterned) modes of GH secretion in putatively low-somatostatin milieu in women." *AM J Physiol Endocrinol Metab*. 297(2) (2009): E483–9.

265. Rosenfeld, Ron G., and Vivian Hwa. "The growth hormone cascade and its role in mammalian growth." *Horm Res*. 71 Suppl 2 (2009): 36–40. DOI: 10.1159/000192434.

266. Spiliotis, Bessie E., et al. "The insulin-like growth factor-1 (IGF-1) generation test as an indicator of growth hormone status." *Hormones (Athens)* 8(2) (2009): 117–28. DOI: 10.14310/horm.2002.1228.

OTHER BOOKS
BY DR. SELMA RASHID

Hormones Explained: Anti-Aging Medicine, Bioidentical Hormone Replacement, and the Controversies

ABOUT THE AUTHOR

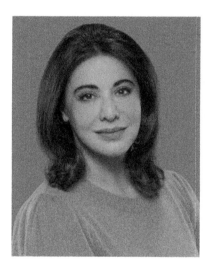

Dr. Selma Rashid was born and raised in England. Trained in Chicago, IL and board certified in Internal Medicine, Dr. Rashid is an expert with over two decades of experience in bioidentical hormone replacement therapy. She works as a hospital physician and is founder and president of the Anti-aging Medical Group. Dr. Rashid is the author of *Hormones Explained: Anti-aging Medicine, Bioidentical Hormone Replacement, and the Controversies*, published in 2010.

Dr. Rashid can be reached at: AntiAgingMedicalGroup.com

Made in the USA
Las Vegas, NV
25 March 2023

69659676R00128